A Crunchy Mom's Hands on Guide to Pregnancy

Dr. Brenda Fairchild, DC, CACCP
and
Elizabeth MacDonald

This book is dedicated to my amazing husband Joe and my beautiful daughter Madelyn. Without them my life and practice would not be what it is today. My pregnancy and delivery took me on this journey to help find answers and help to educate my patients to achieve the birth they want and deserve. I wish I had known then what I know now! I hope you find the book educational and informing to guide you through your pregnancy.

-Brenda Fairchild, DC, CACCP

To all of my children, you have bettered my world and freed my soul. Emmett, my second born, you led me down the path of research and unleashed a passion that I never knew I had.

-Elizabeth MacDonald

DISCLAIMER

This book is to provide you with information and accurate research to help you make an informed choice during your journey of pregnancy.

You should never self-diagnose, and you should always work with your OBGYN, midwife, nurse practitioner, naturopath, and chiropractor.

Also, remember surprises can arise, so having a good relationship and communication with your birth worker is of the utmost importance.

Foreword

Fairchild and MacDonald present a refreshing approach to understanding the importance of a healthy pregnancy, labor/delivery and what to expect post-natal for both you and your baby. Step by step they provide the layperson with an abundance of knowledge to assist you in making healthier choices for you and your baby; laying out the importance of nutrition, exercise, and avoiding stress while building a strong birth team.

Dr. Fairchild further introduces the reader to how to improve the quality of your pregnancy with the knowledge that healthier biomechanics of the pelvis and a more optimal functioning nervous system via chiropractic care is a must for progressive parents.

A healthy and natural pregnancy and birth has been, and always should be, the choice of future parents; and Fairchild and MacDonald have done a tremendous service to help you make informed choices supported by current research.

If there was a must read for those considering pregnancy, I

would put Crunchy Mom's Hands on Guide to Pregnancy at the top. And I will be advocating this book for my patients in my practice.

Claudia Anrig, D.C.

Co-editor, Pediatric Chiropractic

International recognized authority in Prenatal and Pediatric

CONTENTS

Acknowledgments   i

PART 1
What Your Doctor May Not Tell You

1	Importance of Chiropractic Care	Pg 1
2	Prenatal Nutrition	Pg 10
3	Gut Health	Pg 17
4	Supplements	Pg 23
5	Dangers of Common Medications	Pg 35
6	Effects of Stress on Pregnancy	Pg 39
7	Prenatal Exercise	Pg 44
8	Boost the Immune System	Pg 53
9	Pregnancy Ailments	Pg 59
10	Food Cravings	Pg 78
11	Sex During Pregnancy	Pg 89

PART 2
The Breakdown of Labor

12	The Amazing Uterus	Pg 97
13	The First Trimester for the Mom	Pg 102
14	The First Trimester for the Partner	Pg 110
15	The First Trimester for the Baby	Pg 114
16	The Placenta	Pg 121
17	The Second Trimester for the Mom	Pg 125
18	The Second Trimester for the Baby	Pg 130
19	Testing for Gestational Diabetes	Pg 136
20	Managing Gestational Diabetes	Pg 141
21	Sonograms and Ultrasounds	Pg 148
22	The Third Trimester for the Mom	Pg 155
23	The Third Trimester for the Partner	Pg 164
24	The Third Trimester for the Baby	Pg 169
25	Breech Babies	Pg 173
26	Group B Strep	Pg 177

Part 3
Labor

27	Preparing for Labor	Pg 185
28	Relaxation: The Key to Natural Labor	Pg 188
29	The Epidural	Pg 193
30	Family-Centered C-Section	Pg 201
31	Vaginal Seeding	Pg 207
32	VBAC	Pg 211
33	Medical Induction	Pg 216
34	Naturally Inducing Labor	Pg 220
35	Labor Extremes	Pg 226
36	1st Stage of Labor	Pg 231
37	2nd and 3rd Stages of Labor	Pg 243
38	The Placenta After Birth	Pg 246
39	Medical Interventions	Pg 252
40	Labor Complications	Pg 260
41	P.R.O.M.	Pg 267
42	P.P.R.O.M.	Pg 271
43	Preeclampsia	Pg 274
44	Failure to Progress	Pg 279
45	Suctioning at Birth	Pg 283
46	Delayed Cord Clamping	Pg 287
47	Eye Ointment	Pg 292
48	Vitamin K Options	Pg 294
49	Planning a Homebirth	Pg 298
50	Writing Your Birth Plan	Pg 302
	Bibliography	Pg 311

"To be pregnant is to be vitally alive, thoroughly woman, and distressingly inhabited. Soul and spirit are stretched – along with body – making pregnancy a time of transition, growth, and profound beginnings." -*Anne Christian Buchanan and Debra K. Kingsporn*

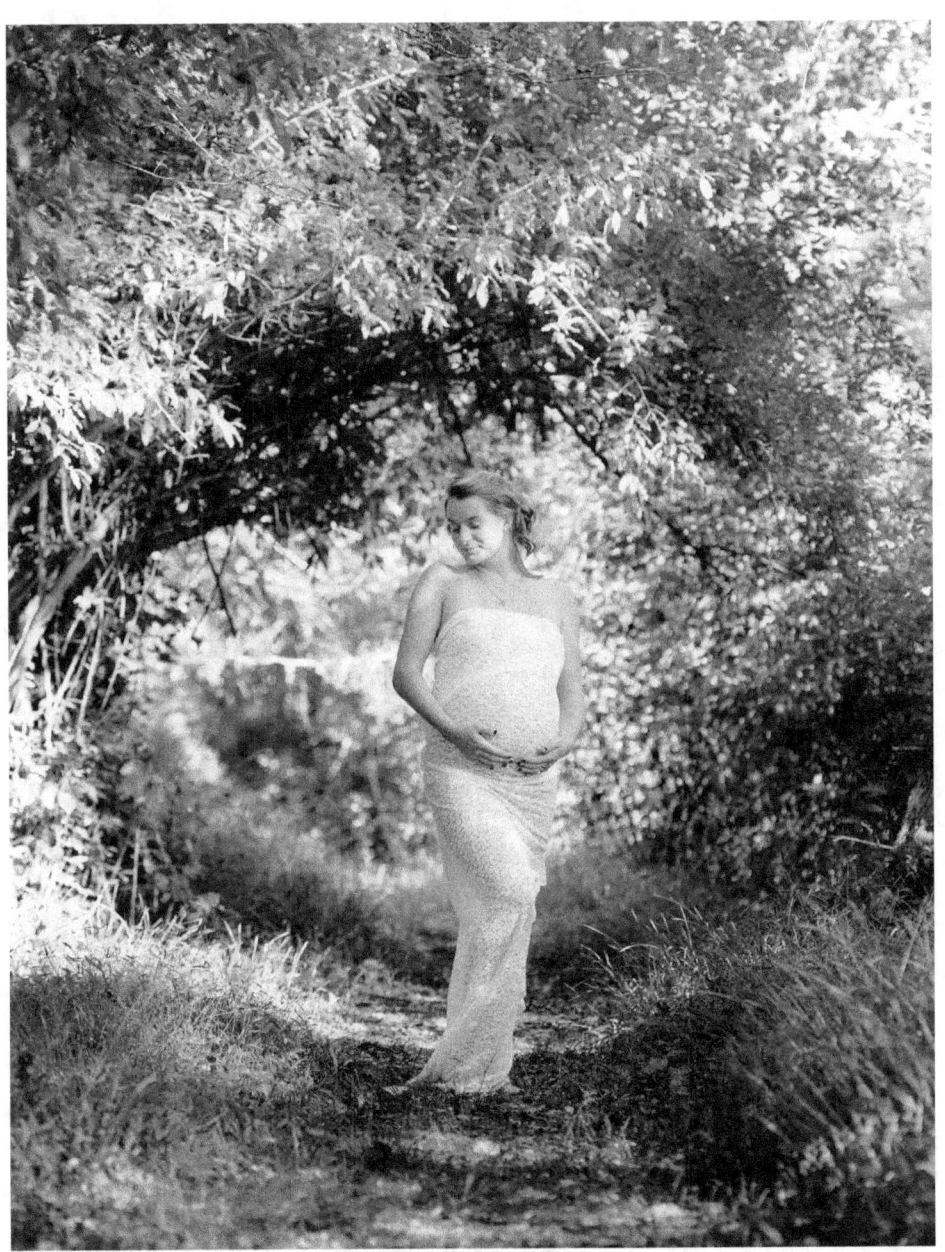

SilverPixels Photography

It is of utmost importance that I begin this book with the Committee on Ethics of American Congress of Obstetricians and Gynecology's view on informed consent.
According to the *second edition, 2004 Ethics in Obstetrics and Gynecology*:

"Informed consent is an ethical concept that has become integral to contemporary medical ethics and medical practice. In recognition of the ethical importance of informed consent, the Committee on Ethics of the American College of Obstetricians and Gynecologists (ACOG) affirms the following eight statements:

1. Obtaining informed consent for medical treatment, for participation in medical research, and for participation in teaching exercises involving students and residents is an ethical requirement that is partially reflected in legal doctrines and requirements.

2. Seeking informed consent expresses respect for the patient as a person; it particularly respects a patient's moral right to bodily integrity, to self-determination regarding sexuality and reproductive capacities, and to support of the patient's freedom to make decisions within caring relationships.

3. Informed consent not only ensures the protection of the patient against unwanted medical treatment, but it also makes possible the patient's active involvement in her medical planning and care.

4. Communication is necessary if informed consent is to be realized, and physicians can and should help to find ways to facilitate communication not only in individual relations with patients but also in the structured context of medical care institutions.

5. Informed consent should be looked on as a process rather than a signature on a form. This process includes a mutual sharing of information over time between the clinician and the patient to facilitate the patient's autonomy in the process of making ongoing choices.

6. The ethical requirement to seek informed consent need not conflict with physicians' overall ethical obligation of beneficence; that is, physicians should make every effort to incorporate a commitment to informed consent within a commitment to provide medical benefit to patients and, thus, to respect them as whole and embodied persons.

7. When informed consent by the patient is impossible, a surrogate decision maker should be identified to represent the patient's wishes or best interests. In emergency situations, medical professionals may have to act according to their perceptions of the best interests of the patient; in rare instances, they may have to forgo obtaining consent because of some other overriding ethical obligation, such as protecting the public health.

8. Because ethical requirements and legal requirements cannot be equated, physicians also should acquaint

themselves with federal and state legal requirements for informed consent. Physicians also should be aware of the policies within their own practices because these may vary from institution to institution."(25)

This means that you have the right to agree to or deny any procedure. Never feel as though you are not a decision maker during this pregnancy. Please use this book as a guide to educating yourself about pregnancy and birth, but I encourage you to dive deeper and learn as much as you can about what is taking place within your body, and all of the possible things that can take place to your body and your baby's body. Knowledge is power. Knowledge is the key to making the best decisions for you and your baby.

Pregnancy

It is sad that most couples spend more time planning their baby registry than their birth. More time is spent organizing a nursery than understanding and learning about pregnancy. This is not the time to blindly trust anyone -even a doctor, who is trained to find problems not support the normalcy of pregnancy.
Before we get into all of the science, research, and education of pregnancy, let's start with the most popular question:
"What should I expect during pregnancy?"

The day you find out you are pregnant, is unlike any other day. The emotions rollercoaster their way into your life: Excitement, Fear, Anxiety, Doubt, Panic, Joy.

You have, on average, 41 weeks to grow this baby. There are no do-overs and you can only do as well as you know to do. Do not feel guilt toward anything up to this point, instead, start today to work toward the best pregnancy you can have.
It is time to learn what will change, how life will be different, and what you can do to help prepare for the birth of your baby; especially if you are walking this path with a natural mindset.

weeks

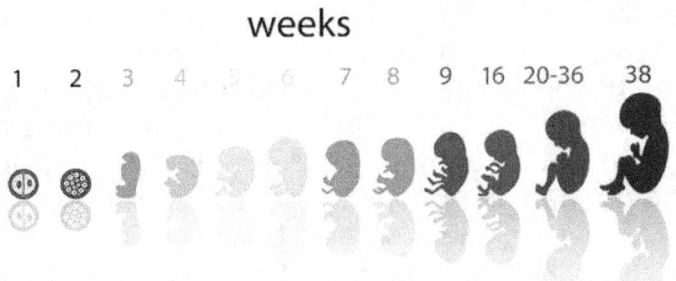

1 2 3 4 5 6 7 8 9 16 20-36 38

The breakdown of pregnancy:

Weeks 1-2

As you have probably noticed, the first two weeks are freebies that the medical community throws in. This is because doctors and midwives base your estimated due date 40 weeks from the start of your last menstrual cycle. If you know your exact date of ovulation, you can calculate your estimated due date by counting 38 weeks from there. However, the average pregnancy is 41 weeks and 1 day in length and is still normal at 42 weeks. So instead of circling a specific day on the calendar, give yourself a "due month," a 4-week window (weeks 38-42) of when baby can make his or her appearance. This will take a lot of weight from your shoulders, and keep people from nagging you once you hit 39 weeks.

Weeks 3-4

Even weeks 3-4 of pregnancy go overlooked to most women, as their period has not been missed yet and most early pregnancy signs can be confused with PMS signs. However, if you were charting your basal body temperature, taking ovulation tests, or hoarding inexpensive pregnancy tests then you may have found out the wonderful news as early as 3 weeks along.

Week 5

Month two begins at week 5. It is a bit early to shout your pregnancy from the roof tops, unless you just can't wait – then shout away! Many women wait until they have heard a heartbeat or enter the second trimester to share, but there are no rules to pregnancy announcements. Your little embryo is rapidly forming, looking quite like a tadpole. Your hCG hormone (human chorionic gonadotrophin) is rising at a very fast rate. This hormone is created by the cells working to form the placenta, and it is to blame for any early pregnancy symptoms you are experiencing.

Weeks 6-12

Between weeks 6-12, you may (or may not) experience a plethora of symptoms. Morning sickness is the most well-known symptom, but don't let the title fool you, it can occur at any time of the day. I will cover the most common symptoms with possible resolutions in chapter 9. Some of these symptoms include:

- Increase in Urination
- Exhaustion
- Breast Tenderness
- Increase in Gas
- Heartburn
- Constipation
- Diarrhea
- Insomnia
- Mood swings
- Fear
- Excitement (1)

Remember that you may have a handful of these or you may have none. Every pregnancy is different.
Not only will you be experiencing a lot during the first trimester, but the tiny growing baby is going through quite a bit as well! I will detail this growth in the upcoming chapters

and talk about just how important the first trimester is for your baby.

Your baby is known as a zygote until week 5, and then an embryo until the 8th week of pregnancy when it becomes a fetus. According to the American College of Obstetricians and Gynecologists (ACOG), the heart and lungs are still developing, and the arms, legs, brain, spinal cord and nerves are beginning to form. By the end of week 8, most of the main organs will have formed. During the third month, weeks 9-12, the tissue which forms bones and muscles begins to grow. The intestines also begin to form and the skin is opaque – almost transparent at this point. It's very important, if possible, to avoid any medications or other harmful items during this stage and all of pregnancy.

Weeks 13-16
The body begins to adjust to the hormones around weeks 13-14, the beginning of the second trimester. This *should* help to level out the intense symptoms, but some women experience them throughout their entire pregnancy. Your belly begins to grow from just bloat to an actual baby bump. Remember that you are only eating for one, and that any extra weight gained from poor food choices means extra weight that will remain after baby arrives.

Weeks 16-20
First time moms report feeling bubbles, flutters, and tiny movements around weeks 16-18 and more intense movements around week 20. If you have an anterior placenta (a placenta that grew on the front of the uterus), movements will be much harder to feel and will not be distinct until later in pregnancy.

Weeks 18-22
Most women elect to receive a 20-week ultrasound during this timeframe. I will cover the pros and cons of ultrasounds and sonograms in chapter 21. If you elect to have the ultrasound, you will learn more than just your baby's gender. Your doctor or midwife will learn:

- placenta placement
- fluid levels
- cervix position
- organ development
- bone length (2)

This is the best time to start preparing for labor. Look into birthing classes, reach out to groups, and start talking birth plans. I highly recommend taking a detailed course on natural childbirth to educate not only you, but your support partner as well.

Weeks 22-27
Hopefully, you have your energy back and are feeling the excitement from each little kick. If you would like, a baby shower, sprinkle, blessing way, or other form of celebration can be planned for the upcoming weeks!

Weeks 28-32
Throughout the third trimester, the enlarged uterus pushes against the mother's diaphragm and causes shortness of breath. Swelling may also occur at this stage, but sudden swelling needs to be discussed immediately with your birth team as it can be early pre-eclampsia.

Weeks 33-36
Welcome to the eighth month of pregnancy! The countdown to full term (now 39 weeks, not 37 like most believe.)(3) has arrived! Baby showers are in full swing, birth classes are happening, books are being read, baby gear is being purchased, and car seats are being installed. Let baby excitement begin!

Weeks 37-40

Your baby is quickly gaining weight, and you may be extremely uncomfortable. Hopefully, baby is head down and engaged for labor, but if not, remember that some babies are still breech or transverse at this point and have the ability to turn before labor begins, and some babies turn once labor begins. Working with your chiropractor can help encourage your baby to find the best birthing position. Braxton Hicks contractions are becoming more frequent and your body may or may not lose its mucus plug. It is hard to be patient these last few weeks, but every day the baby is in the womb and growing means the chances for a healthier baby and labor are increased. Stay positive and let your little one choose his own birthday!

Weeks 41-42

Like how I added in an extra two weeks? Probably not, but it is more common to enter this timeframe then to give birth before 40 weeks. So here you are, being questioned by everyone about when your baby is coming, if you are being induced, and if you are ready for baby's arrival. I suggest you politely let people know that once baby has arrived, you will notify them, but until then – please back away from the belly!

Fairchild and MacDonald

PART ONE

What Your Doctor May Not Tell You

In this section of the book, I will discuss the information that is commonly left out of prenatal visits. I urge you to reach out and interview your birth team to ensure that you feel connected and happy with your selection. *Your birth team should include your biggest supporters.*

Chapter 1
The Importance of Chiropractic Care in Pregnancy

While a chiropractor may not be present at your birth, you can still include them as a member of your birth team. You see, chiropractic care is an essential element of ensuring a healthy and natural pregnancy. it is safe for both mom-to-be and baby. (4)

With our American lifestyle, we are sitting too much and not exercising as much as we should. We are also a stressed out nation as a whole. This is then at an extreme during pregnancy. What exactly is chiropractic care and how can it help have an enjoyable and healthy pregnancy?

The easiest way for me to describe chiropractic adjustments or alignments are that they *help to balance the body*. During pregnancy, as the body is changing and the center of gravity is shifting, the adjustments help to stabilize the spine and pelvis, muscles and ligaments. The alignments help to restore the connection of the spine and the brain (nervous system) along with supporting biochemical/hormonal changes.

There is a specific adjustment for pregnant women called **The Webster Technique.** Discovered by Larry Webster, founder of International Chiropractic Pediatric Association (ICPA) (Where I received my training.), the Webster technique is used every day to help create more space to for the baby to get into a better birthing position. Dr. Webster found that by restoring pelvic neuro-biomechanics, he was able to help breech babies turn into optimal fetal position. (5) Today we call this term in-utero constraint, which I will further discuss momentarily.

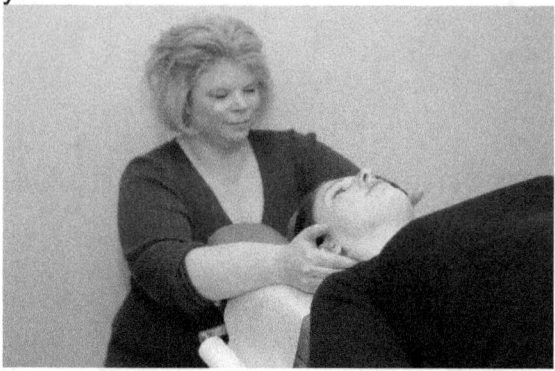

According to the ICPA, *The Webster technique is a specific chiropractic analysis and diversified adjustment. The goal of the adjustment is to reduce the effects of sacral subluxation/ SI joint dysfunction. In so doing neuro-biomechanical function in the pelvis is improved.* When looking for a chiropractor during pregnancy, it is good to make sure they are Webster Certified by the ICPA as these chiropractors are specialized in pregnancy and pediatrics. To find a doctor near you, please visit www.icpa4kids.org.

What exactly is in-utero constraint and why is it important to me? In-utero constraint is defined as 'any forces external to the developing fetus that obstructs the normal movement of the fetus.' Many midwives and some obstetricians know how important fetal position is for the delivery and the well-being of the baby. They can tell a difference between those who have and have not been adjusted. Those who have had their body's aligned typically have a smoother labor and faster birth. When I talk to my 'moms-to-be' in the office, I always say the adjustment is all about the pelvis and sacrum. The uterus and your baby are actually attached to the sacrum with ligaments, so every time you move or the baby moves, it is affecting the biomechanics of your spine.

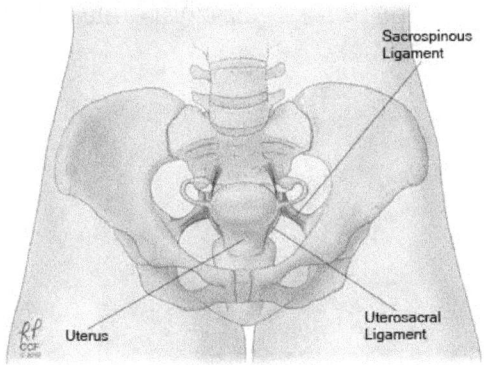

my.clevelandclinic.org/health/articles/pelvic-organ-prolapse/treatment

As your body changes, there can be rotation in the hips and pelvis causing tight muscles which can lead to baby not being in the best position for birth and may cause low back pain or a multitude of different aches and pains that I will be discussing shortly. Not only can this cause pain to you, the mom, but it can hinder the development of the baby in-utero because he does not have the room to develop properly. Here are just a few things that can arise from in-utero constraint to your baby:

- Trouble latching and breastfeeding
- Colicky baby
- Flattening of skull (plagiocephaly)
- Lip tie and/or tongue tie
- Developmental delays
- Torticollis (head tilted or rotated to one side)
- Not sleeping
- Reflux
- Muscles seem tight. Arching back
- Constipation

By utilizing chiropractic care throughout your pregnancy, the specific adjustments to the pelvis, sacrum, ligaments, and muscles will help to keep the maternal pelvis in alignment to allow for your baby to have the most room to develop.

Here are pictures of what a normal pelvis looks like and a pelvis which has rotation.

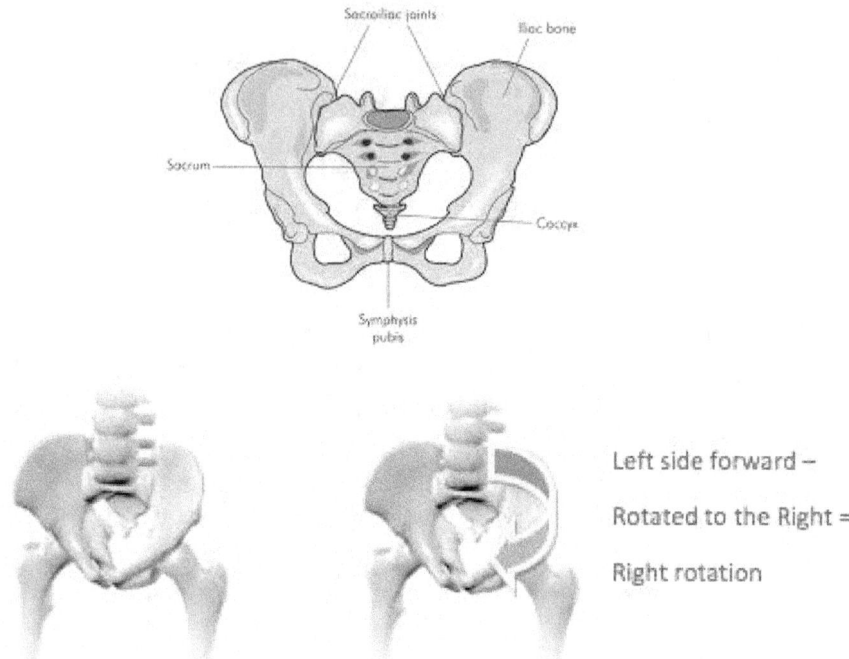

Left side forward –

Rotated to the Right =

Right rotation

As you can see, the pelvic bowl opens generously verses the pelvis with rotation. How does rotation occur? Sitting is the biggest culprit! We sit for hours at a time at work and this makes less room for the baby. Not only does sitting cause intra-uterine constraint, but it causes muscles to shorten and go into spasm, which can lead to neck pain, carpal tunnel, symphysis dysfunction, and low back pain. Other ways that can cause the pelvis to misalign are falls or traumas, stress, biochemistry/vitamins and minerals not being in range, an unhealthy diet, or medications you are taking; all of these may cause the body to be in dis-ease. This is why is it so imperative to see a prenatal chiropractor who can specifically address all of these things with you to help naturally guide you through your pregnancy.

Did You Know?

In a study done by Joan Fallon, chiropractic care helps decrease labor times. Out of the two groups of women who were studies during their first pregnancy, those receiving Chiropractic care averaged 24% shorter labor times than those not receiving Chiropractic care. Of those women who were experiencing their second or third pregnancy, those under Chiropractic care averaged 39% shorter labor times compared to those who were not receiving Chiropractic care. (246)

Chiropractic care not only helps with getting baby into optimal position, but can help with so many aches and pains during pregnancy as well as keeping you healthy as pregnancy can add undue stress on the body over the 9-10 months.
I will detail many of these pregnancy ailments in Chapter 8, but some of the reasons pregnant women come to see me are for:

- Low back pain or Sciatica (shooting pain in legs)
- Neck pain
- Carpal tunnel/numbness and tingling in hands
- Symphysis Pubis Dysfunction
- Headaches
- Numbness in legs

A study involving 400 pregnant women looked at the percentage of women suffering from back pain in pregnancy and whether chiropractic care helped to reduce back pain in labor. Back pain was experienced in 43.5% of pregnancies and 44.7% of the deliveries. Of the 170 pregnancies with reported back pain, 72% also reported back pain during labor. Of the women studied, 37 received chiropractic adjustments during their pregnancies. It was found that 84% of these women reported relief of back pain during labor. (6)

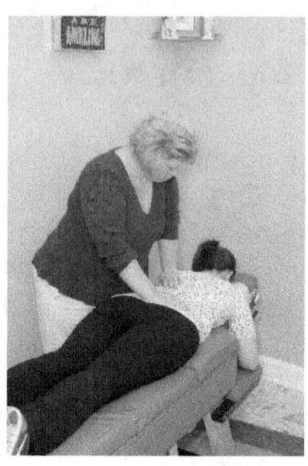

And from my own clinical practice, I have a high percentage of pregnant moms who come in with a lot of back pain and have a wonderful pregnancy without pain and an easier birth with a baby free of dystocia (difficult birth). You should be enjoying your pregnancy and not suffering. Let your prenatal chiropractor help you to enjoy your pregnancy.

Posture

Posture is your window to health! It is everything, and those mammas who have a better posture tend to have a better pregnancy and easier labor. Your posture and center of gravity tend to worsen the further along you go into pregnancy. In my clinical practice I tend to see a shift in posture about every 2-3 weeks. This can be from the baby's position, weight gain, weakening core muscles, increasing breast size causing more rounded shoulder, which leads to neck and head looking downward, tightening hamstring muscles with pubic bone laxity from the relaxin hormone. The poor posture can lead to symptoms such as headaches, neck and low back pain, carpal tunnel, or baby not in optimal position.

To help improve posture when standing, start with knees slightly bent and distribute weight evenly on each leg. I know this will be hard for some of you.

As posture improves, and with continuous stretching of the hamstrings, it will become easier. (Specific exercises will be covered in chapter 7.) Make sure your head and neck are even over your shoulders. Stretching the pec major and minor muscles will help. Try to tuck your buttocks under slightly if you can. This will help to align the pelvis and keep the core muscles stronger.

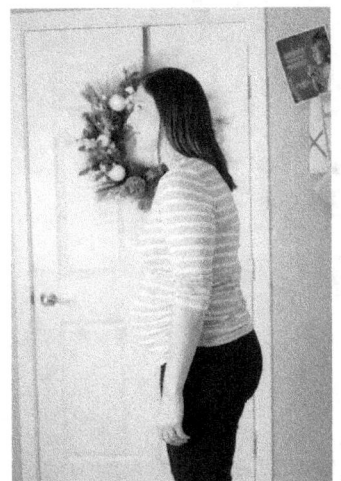

Poor posture

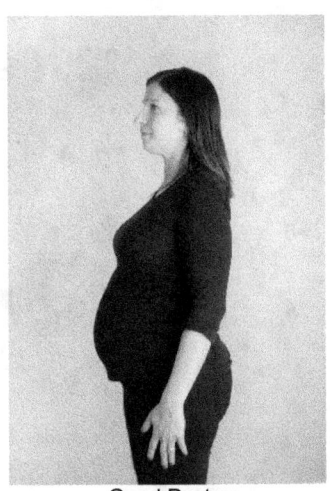

Good Posture

When sitting, I prefer a yoga ball, but if not, make sure your chair has plenty of lumbar support. Make sure head and neck are aligned over the shoulders and abdomen is strong. I recommend you get up and stretch or go for a short walk every 30-60 minutes. This is a great time to stretch the hamstrings and neck and shoulders. This is also a great time to stay hydrated and have a small snack with some protein.

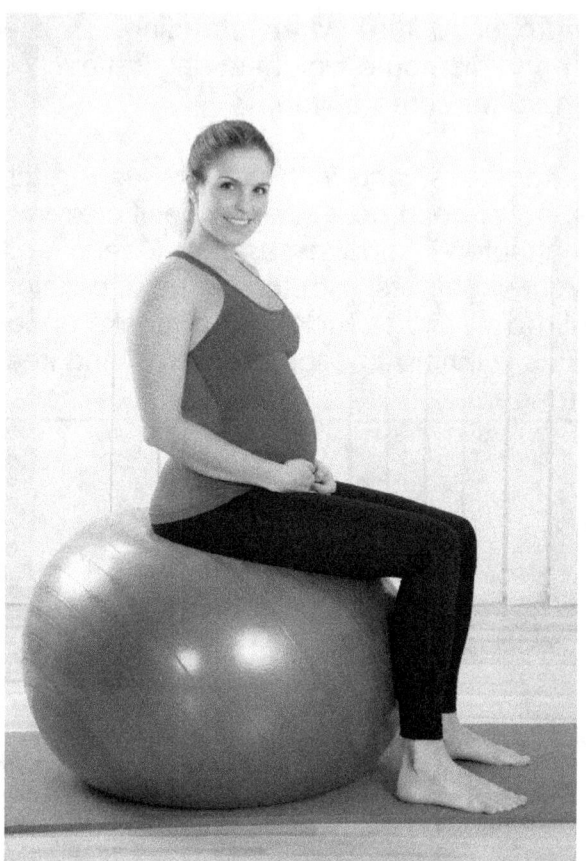

Don't forget, regular chiropractic adjustments throughout pregnancy will help with keeping the body aligned and improve posture.

Prenatal Massage

Chiropractic and massage go hand in hand. Those that get both aligned and massaged feel better longer. Muscles and ligaments are attached to bones, so massages and body work are essential to your prenatal care. According to the American Pregnancy Association, some of the benefits of prenatal massage include relieving muscle aches, decrease swelling, help with anxiety and depression, helping with hormone regulation, and improving sleep.

It is important for you to do your research and find a masseuse that is trained in prenatal massage, not everyone is specifically trained.

Chapter 2
Nutrition: The Key to a Healthy Pregnancy

Deciding on what to eat while pregnant can be mind-numbing. Some foods taste delicious and others make you sick. It is common for women to crave or be turned off by specific foods while pregnant. As you will learn, the placenta is not a filter, but a sponge. It cannot weed out the "good" from the "bad" foods, but instead passes it all to baby. Throwing out the junk and holding yourself accountable during pregnancy will pay off! Eating a well-balanced diet will help you feel better, gain less weight, and increase your chances at a natural birth.

Pregnancy is not the time to go on a diet to lose weight. This could potentially affect the health of you or your child in a negative way. I highly recommend the Brewer's Pregnancy Diet to all of my patients. By following the recommended high-quality protein amounts and focusing on increasing the intake of vegetables and healthy fats (and removing processed foods full of sugars), you will be benefiting your health and the health of your baby. (9)

A well-balanced diet includes foods from all food groups, but pregnancy demands a high ratio of protein to other food categories. This nutrition is essential for normal organ development and functioning, reproduction, and growth. It is needed for resistance to infections and for the ability to repair damage, including reducing the chances of neural tube defects and orofacial clefts. (8)

While pregnancy is a normal condition for the female body, it is stressful, and all nutritional requirements are increased in order to meet the needs of the pregnancy. This does not mean you are eating for two; it means that your food selection is important to obtain the highest quality nutrients!
Instead of portioning and calorie-counting, consume real foods that include as many of these nutrients as possible:

- **Calcium**, to support strong bones and helping to prevent preeclampsia. (27)
  - o Sources: dairy, dark leafy greens, okra, and fish bones
- **Choline**, which is vital for brain development, cell membrane formation and protecting against neural tube defects. (28)
  - o Source: eggs
- **DHA** is essential for your baby's brain formation, as well as eye, skin and nervous system development. (29)
  - o Sources: wild caught fish
- **Folate** (not folic acid) is needed for healthy development and helping to prevent brain and spinal cord defects. (You want to be sure you get the right form if you have the MTHFR defect.) (30)
  - o Sources: dark leafy greens, asparagus and broccoli
- **Iodine** is necessary for the growth of the thyroid hormone. (31)
  - o sea vegetables, cod, shrimp and baked potato with skin

- **Iron** helps builds the placenta and supports oxygenating blood for a growing baby. It reduces the risk of low birthweight and prevents anemia in the mothers. (32)
  - Sources: red meat and liver.
- **Potassium** helps keep the mother's blood pressure in a healthy range. (33)
  - Sources: coconut water, bananas, and avocados.
- **Magnesium** helps the mother sleep and prevents restless leg syndrome, body pain and muscle cramping. (34)
  - Sources: leafy greens, avocados, and brown rice
- **Vitamin A** is essential for baby's brain formation as well as eye, skin and nervous system development. (35)
  - Sources: cod liver oil, liver, and orange vegetables.
- **Vitamin C** helps to keep the bag of waters from rupturing early, and aids in a healthy, full-term pregnancy. (36)
  - Sources: fruits and vegetables.

- High quality *protein* (75 grams or more a day)* helps increase blood volume and prevent anemia. (37)
  - Sources: (local, unprocessed, organic, free-range) grass-fed meats
- High quality *fat* is needed for optimal brain development and nutrient absorption. (38)
  - Sources: coconut oil, organic butter, and nuts & seeds.

Did You Know?

A high protein diet is essential to help avoid pre-eclampsia. You should be eating upwards of 75-120 grams of protein per day. That is the same as 4 chicken breasts. It is a lot, but completely doable! For more information, you can check out The Brewer Diet @ http://drbrewerpregnancydiet.com/index.html

During pregnancy, I have used and have watched many others choose this pregnancy diet, and we all have wonderful things to say about it!

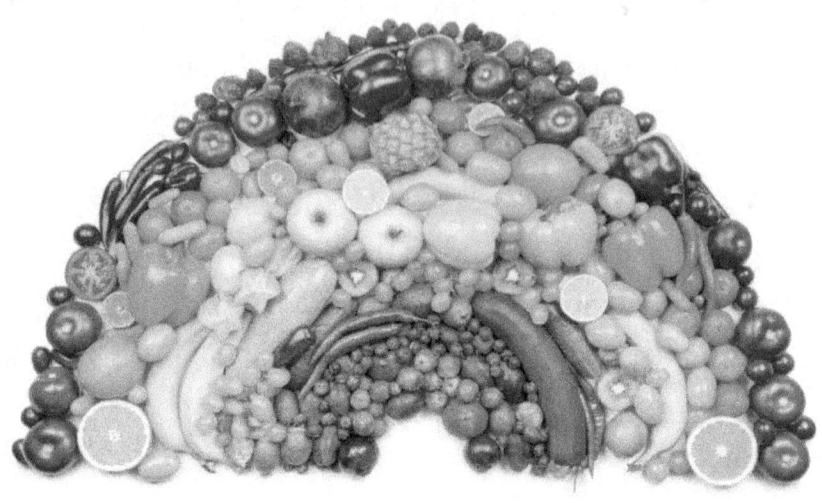

Eat the Rainbow

The easiest way to ensure proper nutrients are being eaten is to include colorful foods: Eat The Rainbow!

The colors come from the different phytonutrients the food contains. So the more colors you consume, the better. Eating this way before and during your pregnancy can drastically reduce the risk of birth defects. (8)

Some women find it hard to transition to a healthier diet, but you can do it. Choose to eat smaller portions more frequently throughout the day so you never reach the point of being overly hungry. You can keep small snacks packed away for easy pick-me-ups (I suggest Brazil Nuts, they contain selenium, which helps with thyroid health.) Remember that low blood sugar can cause problems (and make you grouchy), so keep those healthy snacks on hand. If you are waking up during the night, store an easy-to-grab snack on the bedside table – you will feel happier in the morning because of it.

Wonderful Foods to Include During Pregnancy
(non-gmo, local and organic if possible)

- *Beef and organ meats*
- *Poultry*
- *Eggs*
- *Wild-Caught Seafood*
- *Green Leafy Vegetables*
- *Vegetables*
- *Fruits*
- *Coconut (and Coconut Oil)*
- *Nuts (Peanuts are not nuts)*
- *Bone Broth*
- *Kefir*
- *Whole Grains*
- *Pasture-Fed Butter*
- *Sweet Potatoes*
- *Full-Fat Dairy*
- *Chia Seeds*(7)

Foods Recommended to Avoid

- *Alcohol*
- *Raw fish*
- *Lunchmeats*
- *Raw or undercooked beef or poultry*
- *Unpasteurized juices*
- *Raw dairy*
- *Soy*
- *Legumes*

Soy and legumes have been studied and questioned to be linked to long-term developmental problems in children if consumed by the pregnant mother. While more research needs to be done, I recommend you use your best judgement, and eat organic if you choose to consume these. (39) (40)

Some foods on the above list can be contaminated or hazardous. Foodborne illnesses can include Listeria Monocytogenes, high mercury or lead levels, E. coli, pathogens, parasites, toxicity, and more.

That being said, infection from foods is extremely rare. Talk to your midwife or doctor and do your own research when it comes to choosing foods to avoid.

Non-Foods to Avoid

- *Artificial sweeteners*
- *MSG or chemical additives(41)*
- *Vegetable Oils and trans fats*
- *BPA and plastic containers*
- *Aluminum*
- *High fructose corn syrup (under all of its sudo-names) (42) (43)*
- *Artificial dyes or colors in food*

CHAPTER 3
Gut Health: The Link Between Mother and Baby

Research is now showing that we may be wrong to believe that the womb is a completely sterile environment. Science is showing that the gut bacteria from the mother is able to reach the baby through the placenta.

Our current lifestyle is not very bacteria friendly, and most of us have an imbalance in our gut flora. This imbalance and too much of the 'wrong' bacteria have been linked to premature rupture of membranes (PROM) and premature birth. Science is also linking gut health to chronic illnesses now. (10) (11) (12) (13)

Over 80% of the immune system is in the gut. Therefore, gut health contributes to proper immune function.

The gut controls so much of our bodies – and our health. The gut can signal inflammation to other parts of the body and, if in an inflamed state, can predispose us (and our babies) to everything from autoimmune disease, allergies, asthma, skin problems like eczema and psoriasis to depression, anxiety, symptoms of autism, metabolic problems like obesity, and many neurological problems. (44) (45)(16)(17)(18)

An unhealthy gut is a toxic environment. This toxicity flows from the gut throughout the body and into the brain, which challenges the nervous system. The nervous system is then prevented from performing its normal functions. This is another reason why chiropractic care is so important during pregnancy, as the alignments help to regulate the nervous system.

During pregnancy, your *microbiome* (also known as gut flora) is not only crucial for your health, but for your baby's health as well.

A study sampled stool from pregnant women during each trimester of pregnancy and analyzed the bacteria present. They found that healthy bacteria decreased over the course of pregnancy, while bacteria associated with diseases generally increased. In addition, signs of inflammation in the gut increased.

You would think that these changes would negatively affect the mother and baby, but in pregnancy, they actually trigger changes to the body that aid in energy storage to help the baby grow! (14)

Isn't it amazing how our bodies work?

It is important to build and maintain as healthy of a gut as possible before and during pregnancy. As the flora is altered during each trimester, it will have the strong foundation in which it began.

If you suspect your gut health is not up to par, or antibiotics are needed before or during pregnancy, you can work on repopulating the gut with 'good' bacteria through probiotics and cutting out any inflammatory foods.

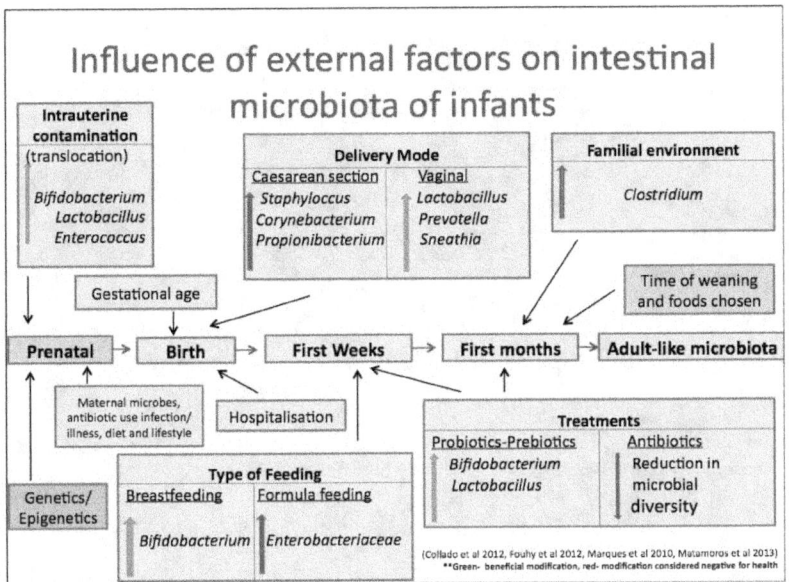

We now know that gut bacteria is transferred to the baby while still in the womb, but there is another process the baby goes through as he is born. "Seeding" is when the mother's bacteria is passed to the baby as he passes through the birth canal and into the world. I will talk more about that further in the book.

Did You Know?

Research now shows that the gut health of the mother effects the brain development of the fetus as early as the first trimester.

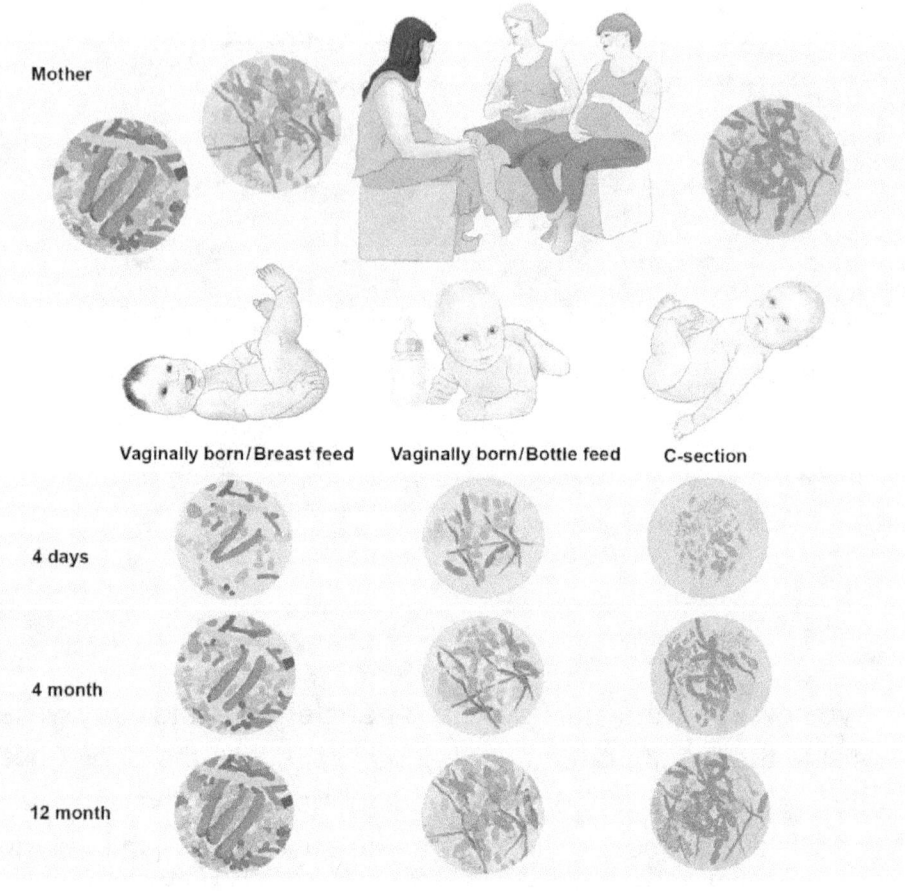

Bäckhed et al./Cell Host & Microbe ---- https://ww2.kqed.org/futureofyou/2016/01/07/dannon-wants-to-make-your-gut-healthy-starting-the-day-youre-born/

Research has also linked symptoms of autism to an abnormal composition of the microbiome. As autism becomes an epidemic in our culture, it is vital to take utmost care of our guts while pregnant, and work to heal any damage.

While you may not be able to avoid all toxic exposures, it's important to reduce your exposure to toxic elements.

20

Unnecessary drugs and vaccinations are two avoidable toxins you can easily decline.

Other ways to avoid toxins include: (19)

1. Buying and eating organic produce and free-range, organic foods.
2. Taking probiotics or working toward healing the gut through diet.
3. Exercising regularly throughout your pregnancy. Research shows that exercise is associated with a significantly higher incidence of vaginal delivery and a significantly lower incidence of cesarean delivery, with a significantly lower incidence of gestational diabetes mellitus and hypertensive disorders. (46)
4. Store your food and beverages in glass rather than plastic – especially if reheating in the microwave.

5. Use natural cleaning products in your home. Vinegar and baking soda are your friends!

6. Minimize stress.

7. Stop smoking.

"A baby is like the beginning of all things: wonder, hope a dream of possibilities. In a world that is cutting down its trees to build highways, losing its earth to concrete, babies are almost the only remaining link in nature, with the natural world of living things from which we spring." – Eda J. Leshan

CHAPTER 4
Supplements for Pregnancy

Prenatal vitamins and supplements. You know you need to be taking them, but it can be a bit overwhelming to choose the right ones.

As I always say, and I have said in my first book, *spend some money and get a great product*. Do not buy over the counter, at a big box store, as many of the supplements are full of fillers(20)

You should go with a reputable company like Klaire Labs, Apex Energetics, Thorne, DaVinci, Seeking Health, Nordic Naturals, Designs for Health, or Standard Process (to name a few). These are some of the best supplement companies out there and their products are made without fillers or dyes and are highly regulated to maintain a superior quality. Most of the products are gluten, dairy, soy, and nut free as well. You will be spending around $20-50 on a good multivitamin. You get what you pay for.
These are the supplements I recommend to take while pregnant. Keep in mind, knowing your specific levels allows you to supplement accordingly:

- Prenatal Vitamin with Folate (not folic acid)
- Omega 3s (Or Fish Oil)
- Vitamin D
- Probiotics
- Magnesium
- B Vitamins
- Iodine
- Chlorella
- Iron

The Prenatal Vitamin

Choosing your prenatal vitamin is one of the most important decisions you can make and choosing should not be taken lightly. The prenatal gummy at the big box store is not cutting it. This goes for many of the multi vitamins that OB's are now prescribing. Remember you are providing nutrients to not only you, but a developing fetus. Provide your baby with the best quality products out there. When choosing a prenatal, the first things I look for are which type of Folate or B9 is listed in the product. Is it Folic Acid (synthetic and found in most supplements, with overdosing linked to cancer (21) and fortified in foods since 1998), Folate (natural in foods), or 5-methyltetrahydrofolate (folate form in supplements)?

Why does it matter?
According to Designs for Health, one of the supplement companies I recommend, Folate is a general term for a group of water soluble b-vitamins, and is also known as B9. Folic acid refers to the oxidized synthetic compound used in dietary supplements and food fortification, whereas folate refers to the various tetrahydrofolate derivatives naturally found in food. Simply put, folic acid is *synthetic* and folate is *REAL*. (22)

Did You Know?

Folic Acid (*not folate*) is linked to: (47)(48)(49)(50)
- Anemia
- Lip and tongue tie
- Birth defects, the most common being spina bifida
- Increased risk of certain cancers

Though the recommendation for pregnancy is 400-600mcg of folate/folic acid, this is the minimal amount recommended. Getting folate from natural sources (spinach, asparagus, turnip greens, mustard greens, parsley, collard greens, broccoli, cauliflower, etc) is always best, but when supplementing for and during pregnancy, you should be taking more than the minimum recommendation. As always, check with a doctor or midwife before taking or changing anything, especially during pregnancy.

Our favorite basic prenatal vitamins are from Thorne and Klaire Labs. You cannot go wrong with either of them.
NOTE: Women who have a MTHFR defect will need to consult with a specialized practitioner and will probably need to take L-5-MTHF which is the methylated form of folate.
Without trying to be too technical, as this topic deserves a book of its own, there is a gene called Methylenetetrahydrofolate reductase (MTHFR) which is part of the methylation cycle to help break down folate.

Some people have this gene mutation and have a hard time breaking down and utilizing folate/folic acid. This can lead to miscarriages and neural tube defects, including lip and tongue tie. I have a lot of moms with anxiety and postpartum depression who are taking extra folic acid. A simple lab test can be done to see if you have MTHFR. I usually recommend the 23andMe genetic profile. https://www.23andme.com/ You will get a ton of information and not just from one gene. For more information, I recommend Dr. Amy Yasko's book *Feel Good Nutrigenomics* to learn more about genes and methylation.

Omega 3s and Healthy Fats

According to the American Pregnancy Association, low intake of omega-3 fats during pregnancy is linked to increased risk of preeclampsia, premature birth and low birth weight. It has also been found to play a role in future hyperactivity in the child. (24)

More recent studies have shown that taking Omega 3 while pregnant may lower the chances of allergies and benefit the cognitive development of your baby. (23)

It's important to realize that your body cannot form omega-3 fats, so a fetus must obtain all of its omega-3 fats from your diet.

Omegas are fatty acids which are crucial during pregnancy. Yes, it is found in your prenatal vitamin, but it usually it not nearly enough and you should be taking extra. Many times you will hear about EPA (eicosapentaenoic acid) and DHA (docosahexaenoic acid). They are important because they help with supporting the brain, heart, nervous system, eyes, and help boost your immune system to keep you healthy.

Approximately 60% of the human brain is composed of fatty material 25% of that material is DHA. Most of us are not eating a diet high in Omega-3's. Add pregnancy into the mix and we tend to become further depleted! After birth, omega-3s are again used to make breast milk, and for women on their second or third pregnancy, levels may be extremely low.

The best source to get your omegas is of course fish, but most fish that is commercially available are polluted with mercury, PCBs and other toxic substances. This is reason enough to include a supplement. Nordic Naturals is one of the best brands around and the gold standard when it comes to omegas. I usually recommend around at least 2000 mg of omegas per day depending on amount of fish consumption.

The last trimester is when your baby's brain development is exploding. Between this brain development and his nervous system both craving DHA, you can understand why I recommend such a high dosage.

Just a reminder, if you plan of breastfeeding you will want to continue to take you omegas due to the baby's brain is developing and needs to be nourished. Please continue to take you prenatal and vitamin D as well.

Did You Know?

DHA has received recommendations from the World Health Organization, the Food and Agricultural Organization of the United Nations and the National Institutes of Health.

Vitamin D

(The Sunshine Vitamin)

I cannot talk enough about vitamin D and its importance of having enough in your body during pregnancy for you and your baby. It is essential for your baby's muscles, ligaments, bones, heart and brain to develop as well as boosting your immunity.

It is VERY important to have your vitamin D levels checked in pregnancy. We know today that levels need to be above 50 ng/ml (Ideally between 60-80) to help protect you and your baby from some of the most serious complications of pregnancy such as premature delivery, preeclampsia, and reduce the risk of diseases such as infantile hypocalcaemia and rickets.

Maintaining optimal vitamin D levels is easily one of the most important approaches you can take to keep both you and your baby healthy.

I follow the Vitamin D council guidelines. **6,000IU** are recommended for moms to be. (51) There are times, depending on lab results, where I may have more or less. If you live in a place where there is a lot of sunshine, you may not have to supplement, verses those of us who live in the Northeast. I prefer a liquid vitamin D as it seems to be more absorbable and people feel better faster. I use the companies Xymogen and DaVinci in the office, but there are others out there as well.

Also, if you choose to breastfeed, research has shown high levels of vitamin D are essential to both you and your baby postpartum. Vitamin D does get into your breast milk! (52)

Did You Know?

Low levels of Vitamin D have been linked to Lower Back Pain. (53)

Probiotics

80% of your immune system is located in your digestive tract, making a healthy gut a major focal point if you want to achieve optimal health!

Gut health is not only vital to your baby's development but sets the tone for the rest of their lives. I want to have the mom free of heartburn and constipation, and try to have her away from antibiotics and acetaminophens during pregnancy. All of these things lower the immune system and change brain chemistry in the fetus. If you have ever heard the gut is your 2nd brain, well it's all true. A healthy gut equals a healthy mom and baby. Poor gut health for mom can lead to a colicky baby, a delay in motor skills and can lead to ADHD later in life. A newborn exposed to unhealthy gut bacteria is also more vulnerable to pathogens, allergens, and a number of immune-related diseases. So getting an infant's gut up and running efficiently is crucial.

Probiotics have been found to:
- Promote a healthy digestive system
- Benefit in treating irritable bowel syndrome and Crones disease
- Strengthen the immune system
- Treat urinary tract infections
- Help in the prevention and management of atopic dermatitis (eczema) in children
- Prevent food allergies in children

During Pregnancy, Probiotics Will:
- Reduce the risk for preeclampsia. Preeclampsia is the number one reason for maternal death in the United States. Probiotics help to reduce inflammation in the intestines, which is believed to lower blood pressure.
- Aid in postpartum weight loss. (54)
- Help digestion and nutrient absorption. Probiotics help to break down proteins, carbohydrates and fats and they convert the fiber into healthy fatty acids that nourish the cells that line the intestinal wall. This can help reduce gas, bloating, heartburn and constipation. The more nourishment you get, the more your baby gets. Probiotics also help the intestines make short-chain fatty acids, which contribute to the overall health of the body.
- Help reduce the risk for postpartum depression. Preliminary research is finding the importance that taking probiotics can alter the neurotransmitters in the gut, boosting the ability to deal and cope with anxiety and depression.

The Standard American Diet needs some help, there's no denying that. Supplementing with a high quality probiotic throughout pregnancy can help rebalance the gut. But choosing a probiotic is not always easy, as there isn't the perfect one out there. You do want to look for something that has 7-10 strands *minimum* of bacteria. I like Davinici and Klaire the best.

A few different strains you may find on labels:
- Lactobacillus acidophilus
- Lactobacillus rhamnosus
- Bifidobacterium lactis
- Lactobacillus casei
- Bifidobacterium Breve
- Bifidobacterium Longum
- Bifidobacterium Bifidum
- Streptococcus thermophiles

Did You Know?

Not only does diet influence your gut (before, during, and after pregnancy), but so does vaginal birth and breastfeeding! (55)

Magnesium

Severe magnesium deficiency can lead to poor fetal growth, preeclampsia, or even fetal death.(56) Proper magnesium levels help mom's tissue growth and recovery during pregnancy and may help baby receive more nutrition through the placenta. I usually recommend 500-1,000mg of magnesium. Everyone is different though. Too much magnesium can cause loose bowels, so that is an easy way to tell if you are taking too much. Typically in pregnancy, many women are constipated, so the magnesium can help you to go on a more regular basis.

I also recommend magnesium oil (a rub, salve, or lotion) on the skin or a magnesium flake foot soak or bath.

Magnesium plays a role in early pregnancy as well as in ensuring a full-term, healthy pregnancy. (15) Magnesium deficiency is all too common in women of childbearing age. It goes undiagnosed and poses many threats to both mother and baby.

Did You Know?

Magnesium can prevent high blood pressure in pregnancy. (57)

B Vitamins

Vitamin B deficiency has been linked to neural tube defects.

It is easy to become deficient, as most women are not getting adequate amounts of B12 in their diets. Consider taking choline along with your B vitamins, as it aids in the proper development of your baby. Research shows that choline is at high demand throughout pregnancy, and together with B12, it helps metabolize folate. (58)

Did You Know?

- Vitamin B6 can aid in alleviating morning sickness.
- Taking a B-Complex Vitamin will cover all your B Vitamins in one.

Iodine

Thyroid hormone demand increases in pregnancy, which requires a good iodine supply that is obtained mostly from the diet or through a supplement. Your baby's thyroid hormone production increases after the first 20 weeks of gestation, which demands more iodine from you. (59)

Iodine can be detected in every organ and tissue in your body. Low iodine levels may be related to numerous diseases, including cancer. It may also severely affect your child's brain, as it is important for healthy brain development. Iodine has been found to boost children's IQ. (60)

Guidelines for daily dietary iodine intake: (59)

Institute	Nonpregnant Nonlactating Adolescents and Adults (µg)	Pregnant Women (µg)	Lactating Women (µg)
Institute of Medicine[48]	150	220	290
WHO, UNICEF, ICCIDD[15]	150	250	250
Endocrine Society[89]	—	250	250

Iron

Having your iron levels checked is standard during pregnancy, but you can request it be monitored to ensure you are meeting your body's needs. You want to make sure you are getting enough, as iron deficiency can cause problems for both you and your baby. Prenatal vitamins with daily iron can

33

reduce the risk of low birthweight, anemia and iron deficiency. (32)

If you have been feeling more tired than normal, consider increasing your iron intake.

CHAPTER 5
Dangers of Commonly Accepted Medications

After revamping your diet and ensuring that your supplements are high quality, there is another step you must consider. Commonly accepted medications, the most popular being acetaminophen, may not actually be safe while pregnant (or when not pregnant – for anyone!).

Acetaminophen has been called into question for decades, but yet remains to be the last remaining member of the class of drugs known as "aniline analgesics" on the market. Acetaminophen only blocks the feelings of pain and reduces fever, it exerts no anti-inflammatory action. In reality, this "pain reducer" can cross the blood-brain barrier and cause inflammation on the brain, all while masking the symptoms.

**But your doctor says it is safe!
So that means that it is safe, Right?
NO.**

You may know this over-the-counter drug as 'Tylenol.'

That's right, acetaminophen is actually dangerous. I'm sure this comes as a surprise to most of you, as most doctors actually recommend this for every ache, pain, and ailment – even during pregnancy. (61)

The International Journal of Epidemiology published a study about children born to mothers who took acetaminophen during pregnancy. The research showed that those who took acetaminophen were more likely to have behavior problems and slow motor development at age 3. (62) JAMA Pediatrics latest research has also concluded children who were followed through 61 months of age had a higher incidence of having behavior problems including hyperactivity and emotional symptoms. (63)

Even scarier than this information is that the U.S. Food and Drug Administration rating system for drugs in pregnancy ranks acetaminophen safer than ibuprofen, and much safer than aspirin. *The truth: There are no "safe" pharmaceuticals to take while pregnant (or at all.)* So much is unknown about fetal development, especially in relation to pharmaceutical drugs. Therefore, every mother should do her best to avoid taking any pharmaceuticals.(64)

The brain is rapidly developing while in utero, and research suggests that acetaminophen is a hormone disruptor. Abnormal hormonal exposures in pregnancy may influence fetal brain development. This is VERY scary. (64) But, because women believe it to be safe, acetaminophen is the most commonly used pain and fever medication during pregnancy. However, the positive link between acetaminophen use and autism spectrum disorders should be enough to make you toss the acetaminophen! Research shows the longer the acetaminophen is used, the higher increased risk of autism for the child or infantile autism with hyperkinetic symptoms occurring. Studies also suggest acetaminophen exposure early in life can impact hyperactivity.

While we are talking about the safety of common medications, I feel responsible to at least mention the danger of vaccinating while pregnant. There has *NEVER* been any research done to prove that it is safe to vaccinate while pregnant. That's correct. Not one paper; not one study. No one has any idea the consequences to you or your unborn child. Most OBGYN's as well as the CDC are now recommending in pregnancy the Flu shot as well as the pertussis or DTap. (65)

So, how do you know they are safe? How do you know if you will be a statistic or not?

I discussed vaccines in my last book, *Why Didn't My Pediatrician Tell Me That?* Here's a little recap on how vaccines actually work. It all has to do with T-helper cells.

T-helper cells are involved in our adaptive immunity. They help us to fight off bacteria and other viruses that we come in contact with. We should have an even balance of Th1/Th2 cells. T helper 1 (Th1) help to fight off bacteria, viruses, and cancers from inside the cells, otherwise known as our cellular immunity. When we are exposed to illnesses such as chicken pox or measles, our body elicits a Th1 response and supposed to give us a lifetime of immunity from chicken pox. We should never get it again.

The T helper 2 (Th2) are activated to fight off extracellular parasites, (including vaccines) and is described as humoral immunity. If there is too much Th1 you can have a delay in skin reactions. If a person has a high Th2 ratio, this can cause symptoms like a constant runny nose, eczema, allergies, and asthma, as well as autoimmune diseases such as hashimotos and lupus. (9) (10). This may sound familiar to some of you.

Vaccinated adults and children tend have a high ratio of Th2 over Th1, which is why some are prone to chronic illness and autoimmunity. There may be a possible correlation to the number of vaccines given during pregnancy and newborns which could be why the US is so high on the chart with infant mortality rates (66)

According to the CIA, in 2015 the infant mortality rate (IMR) in the United states was 5.87 deaths per 1,000 live births and we were ranked 167 in the word. Afghanistan was first with 115/1,000. And the lowest IMR was Monaco at 1.82/1,000 births. Monaco has less vaccines than with the united states has. (67)

According to Organization for Economic Co-operation and Development (OECD) the US spent the most on health care per person with $8,745 per person, yet we have a high IMR and people are getting more sick all the time. (68) So, where do we start to make a change?

Chapter 6
The Effect of Stress on Pregnancy

I know that I've given you a lot to think about already, but stay with me. I want to get everything out on the table, so you are thoroughly informed and can make educated decisions throughout your pregnancy.

Stress is pretty unavoidable, but the lasting effects that it can have on the body – and baby – are reason enough to take up practicing prenatal yoga.

Research shows that stress experienced by a woman during pregnancy may affect her unborn baby as early as the first trimester, with potentially harmful effects on the brain, gut and overall development. (69)

Pregnancy in itself is a stressful time on a woman's body. The normal physical and hormonal changes can be quite daunting, but the reality is that excessive stress during pregnancy can have some severe consequences for the health of an unborn baby if it is not well managed.

It's already known that extreme stress during pregnancy can lead to increased risk of miscarriage in early pregnancy, but in toward the end of pregnancy, extreme stress can lead to premature labor and birth. The latest findings indicate that prenatal stress can also increase the risk of a baby being born with asthma or allergies, and so many other lifelong challenges.

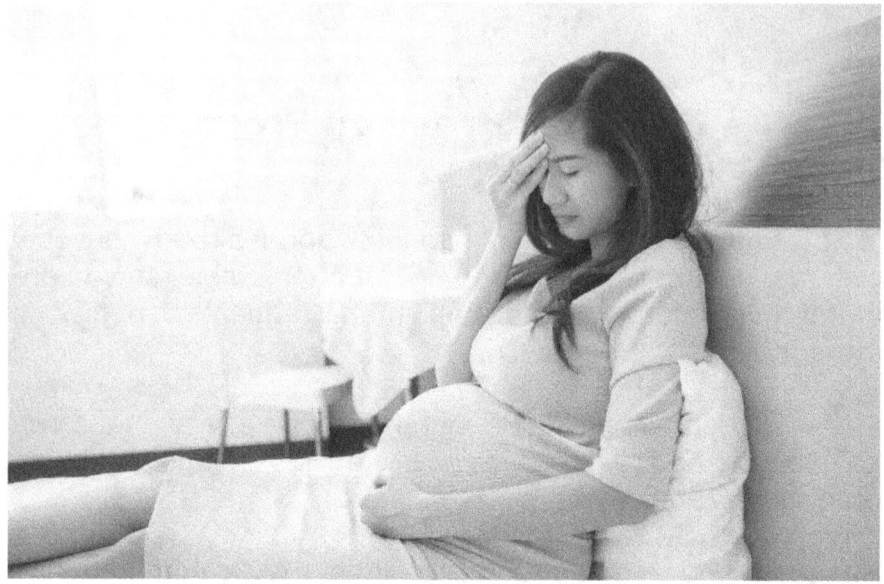

Don't stress out about being stressed, that will be the opposite of helpful. Instead, use this information to eliminate stress triggers in your life.

Women under higher than normal stress levels, chronic stress, or stress that is not handled well are exposing their babies to increased levels of cortisol. These cortisol levels can affect the birth and the baby. You see, cortisol is passed to the baby from the mother through the placenta. (70)

Increased cortisol directly effects the baby's developing nervous system, and it can trigger preterm birth. Several studies have documented that relatively high levels of prenatal maternal cortisol predict: (71)(72)

•   Greater behavioral and physiological stress reactivity in fetuses, infants and children
•   Decreased cognitive ability in infants
•   Increased affective problems in young children
•   Altered amygdala volumes in young girls

Stress during the first trimester of pregnancy alters the population of bacteria living in your vagina. These changes are then passed on to your baby during birth.

According to research presented in 2013 by the Society of Neuroscience, "features of the mother's vaginal microbiome were altered by stress, and in turn, changes were transmitted to the offspring's gut."

Tracy Bale, senior author on the study and a professor of neuroscience in Penn's School of Veterinary Medicine and Perelman School of Medicine states:

'As the neonate's gut is initially populated by the maternal vaginal microbiota, changes produced by maternal stress can alter this initial microbial population as well as determine many aspects of the host's immune system that are also established during this early period.'

This shows just how much of an effect stress has on the baby's gut and brain development.

A study released in March 2015, utilized the information provided by baby's first blood draw (heal prick) after birth, shows that infants whose mother's cortisol levels were consistently higher than normal early on in pregnancy, had higher than normal cortisol levels themselves. (74)

These infants exhibited a much higher sensitivity to stress than other babies with lower cortisol levels. As they grew into toddlerhood, they each had heightened levels of anxiousness compared to other children, and by the time they were six years old, MRI scans revealed their brains were different. The section of the brain associated with the human response to being scared was larger than normal.

Increased stress in pregnancy also elevates the fetal heart rate. Research comparing stress to mood changes shows that a bad mood or bad day does not alter the fetus, but stressful situations and lifestyles do. (75)(76)

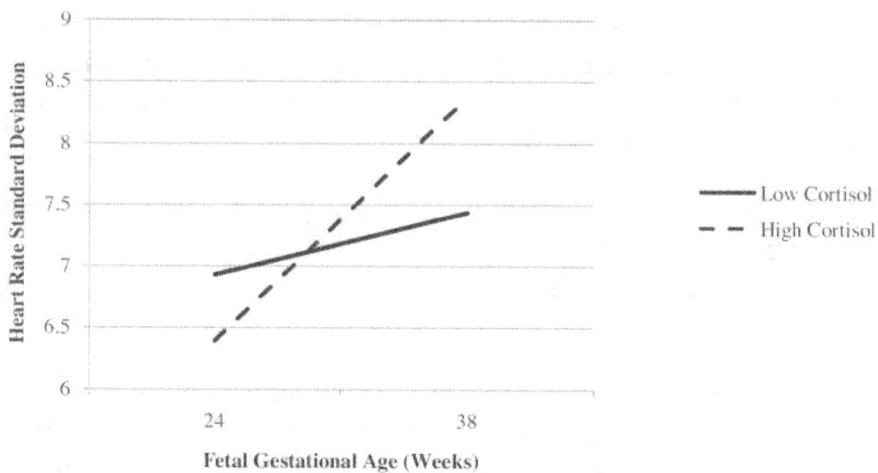

As if stress didn't effect enough, it can also alter your baby's IQ. That's right, maternal stress passed to baby can lower his intelligence and cause attention problems. (77)

As you can see below, your stress can also impact normal tissue and organ development within your baby, and increase the risk of developing of cardiovascular, metabolic syndromes, strokes or various neurobehavioral, neuropsychological, neuropsychiatric diseases later in life. (78)

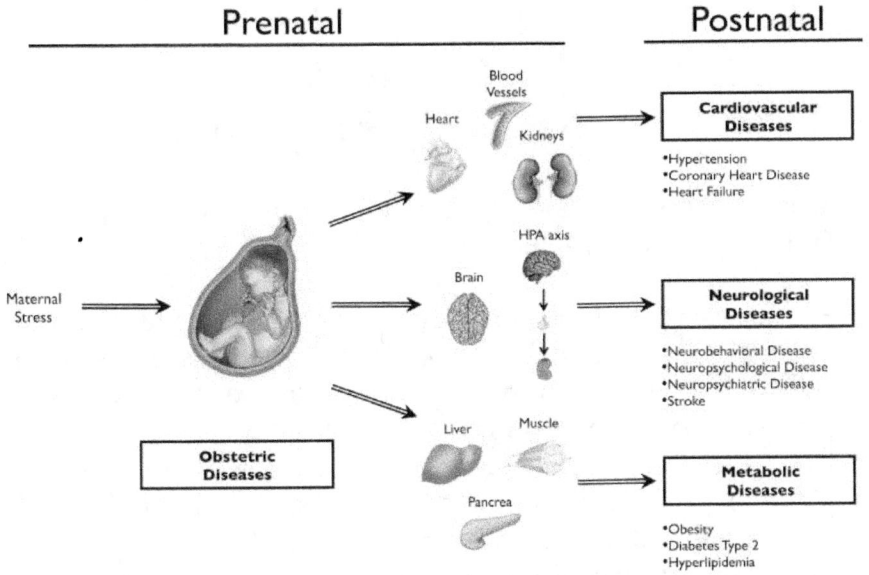

Prenatal

Postnatal

Did You Know?

Stress during pregnancy can also cause: (78)
- Asthma and Allergies
- Cardio-Metabolic Syndrome
- Stroke

The most common forms of stress that pregnant women experience include:
- Relationship Problems
- Work
- Finances

Stress is going to happen. It is inevitable. But how you handle the stress is what is important. Working through it before it becomes ongoing and overwhelming will help lower your chances of any maternal stress-related complications.

Chapter 7
Exercise Myths vs Facts

One of the best ways to conquer stress is through exercise. But what is safe while pregnant?

For some reason, pregnancy is viewed as a medical illness, in which one must carefully walk on egg shells or be criticized by everyone! Why is that? Women have been having babies for centuries. The truth is that pregnancy is the most natural thing a woman's body can take on. If you were living a healthy lifestyle prior to conception it can be continued throughout pregnancy without a second thought, at whatever level you feel comfortable with – But if there is ever a time to take a step toward living healthier, pregnancy is it. (79)

It's time to get moving!

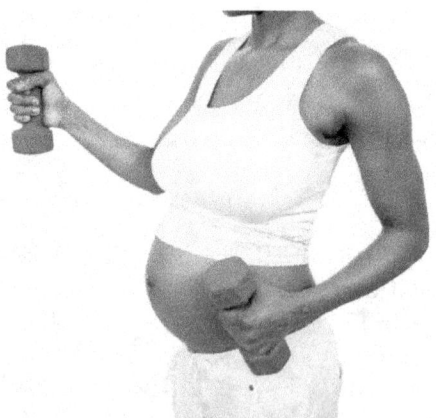

There is a lot of false information circulating on exercising while pregnant. I want to cover the biggest myths, discuss the benefits, and provide some sample exercises for the low-risk, healthy pregnant woman.

According to Raul Artal, MD, lead author of the American College of Obstetricians and Gynecologists' (ACOG) guidelines on prenatal exercise, "nowhere in the medical literature does it say that moderate exercise such as walking is unsafe, even for previously sedentary women." For normal, healthy pregnancies, Artal recommends walking 30 to 60 minutes a day, broken up however you'd like. The ACOG recommends that previously inactive women should start slowly — beginning with as little as 5 minutes of exercise a day and adding 5 minutes each week until they can stay active for 30 minutes a day.

Myths about exercising while pregnant

Exercise increases miscarriage rates: *MYTH.* About 20% of early pregnancies end in miscarriage. Studies show that there is no correlation between low to moderate intensity exercise and miscarriage. According to research, physical fitness appears to be a protective factor of established pregnancies and not significantly involved in the risk of early miscarriage. (80) (81) (82)

Exercising increasing chance of injury: *MYTH.* While, the body does produce more of the hormone relaxin during pregnancy, it has no relation to an increase in injury possibilities. Using good form, and working out correctly will keep you injury free.(83)

Blood Flow is taken from baby: *MYTH.* Exercise promotes an increase in blood flow (and healthier, oxygenated blood) through the body. This actually means that there will be an increase in blood flow to baby, not a decrease!

The womb will overheat: *MYTH.* While overheating can be dangerous to the developing fetus, especially in the first trimester, it is very hard to do. (84) The woman's body is built to grow babies and protect them while in utero. You can feel overheated and dizzy, which means that you should STOP activity. Even at this point, your baby is safe and healthy in a perfectly kept temperature of amniotic fluid. Listen to your body, drink water, and rest when needed. Pregnancy increases blood volume, but allows you to sweat at lower body temperatures, which actually reduces the risk of your body temperature getting high enough to bother the baby. You have an increased ability to get rid of excess heat or store it – the new tissue needs to be 'kept warm.' This allows pregnant women who are physically active to better manage heat stress better than non-exercisers.

The placenta can be displaced or rupture: *MYTH*. Placenta previa cannot be caused by exercise, neither can a rupture. Studies show that exercising provides blood higher in nutrient volume to the placenta, helping to create a healthier supply for baby.(79)

The umbilical cord may become tangled: *MYTH*. The cord may become knotted and twisted throughout pregnancy even if you are confined to your bed. An active baby is the cause of this, not your workout routine.

Exercise can cause a low birth weight for baby or a premature labor: *MYTH.* The length of pregnancy will not be affected by exercise. There is no data showing exercise is linked to low birth weights either.

Walking is enough: *MYTH.* Walking around at a leisurely pace is not enough to count as exercise. Your heart rate needs to increase, breaths quicken slightly, and the body needs to work.

I Have Gestational Diabetes, I can't exercise: *MYTH.* Studies show that exercising while having gestational diabetes poses absolutely no risk to mother or baby. Research states that women with gestational diabetes benefit just as those without do through exercising. (85)

You cannot perform abdominal exercises: *MYTH.* Your abdominals and your entire core, including your pelvic floor, should be strengthened throughout pregnancy, and doing so will help not only during pregnancy, but also in labor, delivery, and recovery. Abdominal exercises also help with posture support, which will benefit you throughout pregnancy and afterward.

Nutrients will be depleted and baby won't get what he needs: MYTH. Baby will get what he needs. Your body will take the nutrients from you, but not your baby. Eat small, frequent meals to keep blood sugar levels balanced.

Your heartrate should not go above a certain point: MYTH. There is no specific target heartrate that suites every pregnant exercising woman. ACOG abandoned the "target heart rate" concept a long time ago. What they and most experts now rely on as a guide is RPE, or rate of perceived exertion.

You can't lie on your back: MYTH. While you should try not to be on your back for long periods of time (like overnight), there is no reason to avoid this position while exercising. The body will cut blood supply to your legs before depriving the baby of anything. You will feel tingling and numbness, dizziness, and nausea if the body needs to move.

Women should not try any new exercise regimen once pregnant: MYTH. There is no research to warrant this claim. If anything, exercises should be added to ensure that working out lasts the entire pregnancy and helps to prevent excess weight gain. If you are a runner, add in the elliptical or bike. That way you have options throughout pregnancy. Adding new strength training exercises is fine as well, using natural body weight is always a great option.(86)

I have to stop after the second trimester: MYTH. Some of the best outcomes associated with exercise during pregnancy occur when fitness continues until the end of pregnancy.

Exercise not only is healthy, but it is good for the soul. I know that it is hard to make time or figure out the right way to start, but I promise that you can do it. If you need to use this pregnancy as your excuse, then go for it!

The Prenatal Benefits of Exercising:
- Lowers excess weight gain
- Increases blood flow
- Reduces pregnancy-related discomforts (87)
- Improves calcium absorption, preventing hypertension, preeclampsia, and future osteoporosis: Studies show that physical activity during the first half of pregnancy is likely to reduce the risk of pre-eclampsia and gestational hypertension. (88)
- Relives tension, stress, and depression
- Increases general strength, improving the ability to carry the baby belly with a strong posture
- Reduces the strain on the upper back
- Reduces the strain and pressure on the lower back and sciatic nerve
- Prevents improper posture
- Improves Sleep
- Increases energy, particularly in the third trimester
- Improves immunity
- Improves self-image and self-esteem
- Provides a sense of achievement
- Provides a positive outlook on pregnancy
- Strengthens, tones, and gives better control of the pelvic floor muscles during labor
- Improves endurance, and muscle control for a less painful labor
- Lowers risk of c-section
- Reduces rates of birth defects
- Increases chances of high APGAR scores for baby (89) (90)

Did You Know?

Exercising while pregnant benefits you after pregnancy. In the short term, studies show that the babies of exercising moms handle the stresses of birth better than babies of non-exercising women.

Postpartum benefits include: (91)
- Minimized stretch marks
- Minimized Baby Blues (92)
- Minimized Urinary Leaking
- Faster Recovery time
- Increases energy
- Improves child's health: Research shows that exercise can prevent the chemical marks on genes that lead to diabetes.
- Improves child's neurological, mental, and physical development

Recommended Exercises

As a chiropractor, I am all for exercising, especially when the exercises are proven to help a specific cause. Pregnancy is not an illness, but a natural event. Pregnancy needs to be acknowledged and accepted as such. Exercising throughout will strengthen the bond with the baby, as well as grant both mother and baby many lifelong benefits.

My co-author, a pre and postnatal exercise specialist, recommends that you speak with a dedicated expert to come up with a tailored workout plan specifically for you. But by really listening to your body, you can figure out what feels right. If you were running pre-pregnancy, keep running. If you were taking yoga, keep training. Trust your body and yourself to know what is right. Drink plenty of water and stop if you feel overheated, dizzy, nauseated, or uncomfortable. (89)

Kegels: The hammock-like muscle of the pelvic floor needs to be toned and strong, or you will not enjoy your postpartum bladder issues. To perform a kegel, you squeeze the muscle you use to control urination. The Mayo clinic recommends holding each contraction for five seconds, and then relaxing for five seconds. You can work up to keeping the muscles contracted for 10 seconds at a time. These should be done as often as possible throughout the day.(93)

Pelvic Rocks: Great for core strength and low back pain, pelvic rocks also encourage baby to settle and engage in a position that is ideal for birth. On your hands and knees, you will slowly contract the abdomen and round the back as high as possible while tucking your chin to your chest. (Like a cat.) then you will exhale as you drop your abdomen toward the floor, arching your back, and looking toward the sky. As you perform pelvic rocks, make sure that you include your pelvis in the exercise. Tuck it under as you round upward and feel it expand as you arch down. (94)

Squats: Squatting strengthens the legs and glute muscles, but it also prepares you to able to birth in the most effective position. Squatting while in labor shortens the birth canal, which can make for more effective pushing and a quicker labor.

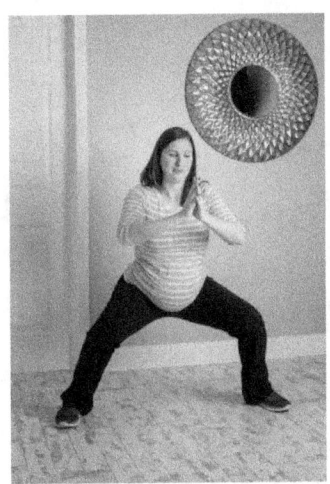 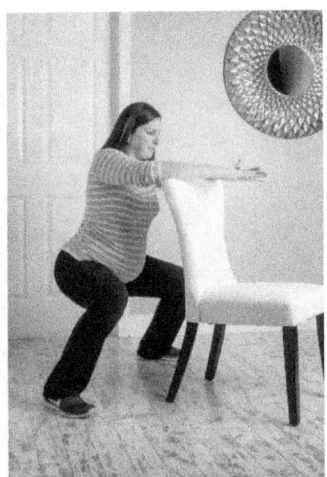

Cardio: Preparing the body for the endurance of labor, cardio gets the heartrate up and the blood flowing. All of that nutritious oxygenated blood is flowing to your baby!

Relaxation/meditation: Not only will this help prepare you for labor, but it can decrease the risk of postpartum depression. (95) (96)

Strength training: Paired with cardio, strength training keeps the muscles toned and able to burn fat, helping to not gain excess weight.

Group classes: Group classes hold you accountable for showing up. Sign up, make friends, sweat, smile, and feel good about yourself.

Stretching/Yoga: Flexibility should be part of everyone's training program, yet it's rarely included. Now is the time. For your flexibility training, do yoga, especially prenatal yoga. A good instructor will help you work on your fitness and your bond with your baby.

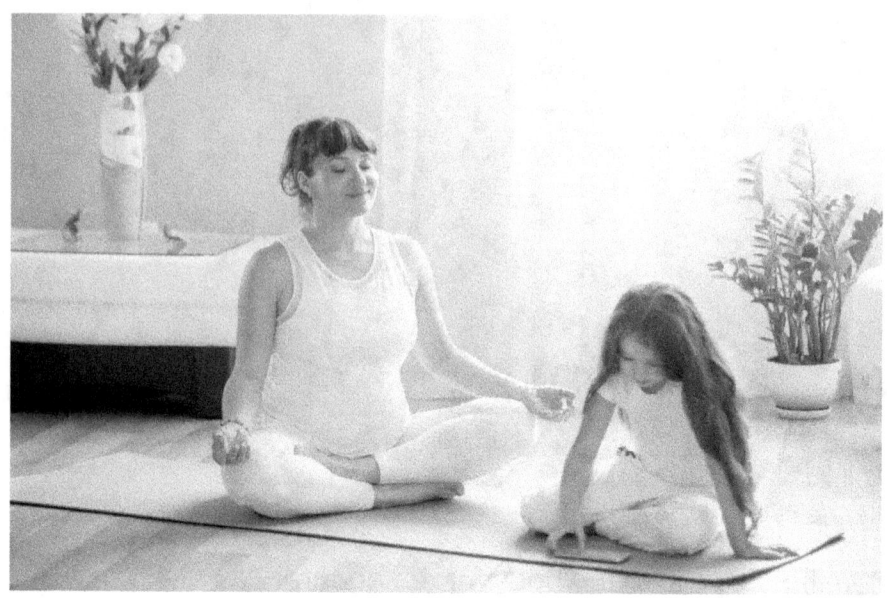

ACOG lists these warning signs to stop exercising immediately and contact a doctor: vaginal bleeding, fluid leaking from the vagina, decreased fetal movement, uterine contractions, muscle weakness, calf swelling or pain, headache, chest pain, increased shortness of breath, dizziness, or feeling faint.

Always talk to your doctor or midwife before beginning something new, or if you have any questions.

Chapter 8
Natural Ways to Boost The Immune System

Now that we have stress under control and an exercise plan in place, it's time to think about boosting your body's ability to fight off illness while pregnant. The immune system is busy protecting the baby, so you may be more susceptible for getting sick.

Try not to wait until you are already sick, but instead work on naturally keeping your immune system ready to fight off illness.

Consider supplements

As you have read, proper, high-quality supplements are important during pregnancy. They may also be taken preventatively to boost the immune system, or as treatment if you are sick. Some that I recommend are as follows:

a. **Vitamin D3** – Vitamin D destroys the cell walls of bacteria, fungi, and viruses, including the influenza virus. (By now you should know that Vitamin D is a must for every aspect of pregnancy – and non-pregnancy!)

b. **Elderberry** - Elderberry is very high in antioxidants and is a good source of potassium, vitamins A, B and C and nutrients like, amino acids, carotenoids, and tannin. (97)

c. **Echinacea** (Not with Goldenseal)–Medical research has shown it to be safe and effective in decreasing the frequency, duration, and severity of common illnesses such as ear and sinus infections, colds, and the flu.(98) (99)

d. **Vitamin C** – This simple vitamin can fight off invading germs and shorten a cold by 19%. (100)

f. **Zinc** – Zinc can help reduce the duration of a cold. (101) (102)

g. **Probiotics** – As you have read, probiotics help to regulate the immune system by balancing the good bacteria (flora) in the stomach. These "good" microorganisms potentially reduce the risk of diarrhea and respiratory infections.

Evaluate Your Diet

A healthy immune system begins with a healthy diet. Yes, this means you will be preparing and cooking more, but grab a crockpot and let it do the work for you. Most foods that boost immune system are those that are good sources of one or two particular vitamins, minerals or nutrients, so eat a wide range of foods.

For the immune system to function properly and be able to defend your body against pathogens, it is very important to supply the body with a sufficient amount of all vitamins, minerals, antioxidants, and amino acids. It is also important to limit or eliminate refined sugar. As you have read, it is basically a poison which, among other things, dramatically decreases immune function.

Foods to Include for Immune Boosting:

Ginger: Ginger contains many bioactive components, helping to decrease oxidative stress markers and boost the immune system. (103)

Pomegranate: Another antioxidant that reduces oxidated stress. (103)

Garlic: It is antibacterial, antiviral, and anti-fungal. Garlic has some serious infection-fighting capabilities! (104) (105)

Bone Broth: Homemade can't be beat! You guarantee all ingredients are high-quality. This is a cure-all in traditional households; bone broth or stock can be made from chicken, fish, or beef bones. It builds strong bones, soothes sore throats and nourishes the soul!

Almonds: Vitamin E is a fat-soluble vitamin, meaning it requires the presence of fat to be absorbed properly. Almonds are packed with vitamin E and provide a prebiotic boost and reduce oxidated stress.

Citrus: Almost all citrus fruits are high in vitamin C, so pick your favorites and enjoy.

Red Bell Peppers: red bell peppers have twice as much vitamin C as citrus, as well as being a rich source of beta-carotene. (106)

Broccoli is super-charged with vitamins and minerals. It is packed with vitamins A, C, and E, as well as numerous antioxidants. Broccoli is one of the healthiest vegetables you can put on your table.

Spinach is full of antioxidants and polyphenols. It can help lower cholesterol and fight off oxidated stress. (107)

Full Fat Yogurt (and Kefir): Probiotic-packed foods!

Mushrooms: Containing beta glucans, mushrooms can positively impact and strengthen the immune system to prevent infections. (108)

Essential Oils

While it is not shown safe to ingest any essential oils, you may diffuse them, use them in salves, rubs, baths, etc. There are "hot" oils that should not be used on children, so make sure you know what you are purchasing and how you are using it.

Exercise

Physical activity may help push bacteria out of the lungs and airways. This can reduce your chance of getting sick. It causes changes in antibodies and white blood cells, which circulate more rapidly and detect illnesses earlier. (109)

Massage

Just what you have wanted to hear! As you have read, prenatal massages have many benefits. They calm you down and even helps you sleep at night.

Sleep

Let the immune system recharge and rest.

Fresh Air and Germs

Yes, you read right – GERMS. Not all germs and bacteria are bad for you! Some exposure to germs can help build your immunity and protect them from illness. As homes become cleaner and more sterile, the immune system doesn't have to work as hard to defend the body against common illnesses. A little dirt won't hurt, if anything, it may help! (110)

Skip The Chemical-Filled Products

Anything you put on the skin is absorbed into the body, either helping or hurting yourself and possibly your baby. From toothpaste to shampoo, read your labels!

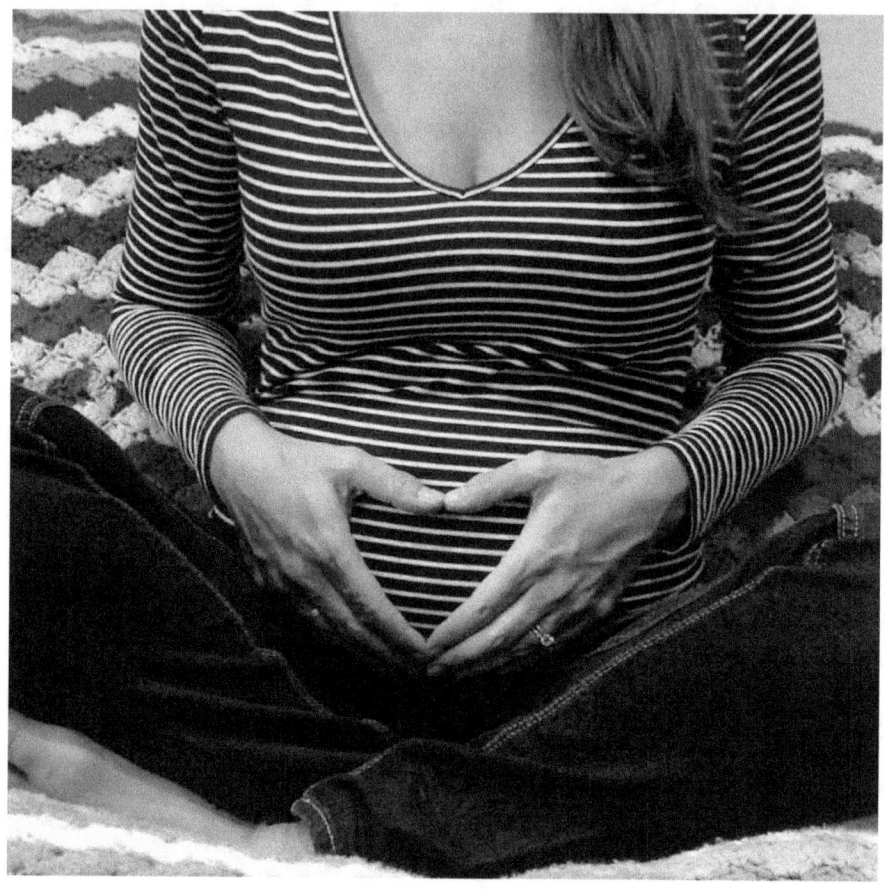

"Everything grows rounder and wider and
weirder, and I sit here in the middle of it all and
wonder who in the world you will turn out to be."
– Carrie Fisher

Chapter 9
Pregnancy Ailments: What's Normal and How to Help

You can be as healthy as physically possible while pregnant and still suffer from pregnancy related ailments. Every pregnancy is different, and whether you are an anxious, high-stressed mom-to-be who wants to know every possible ailment that may be heading her way; or you are a mellow, mom of four who thought she had experienced it all, this chapter may become a useful tool.

It needs to be noted that a woman should always trust her gut. Your birth team should be 100% supportive of you and your needs. They should answer questions and never dismiss your concerns. Although rare, some very normal and common pregnancy ailments may be linked to something that needs medical attention. Do not be shy about speaking up.

It is perfectly normal to have no real symptoms at all. But if you are experiencing ailments, trying to handle them naturally is always the best solution.

Heartburn

Wives' Tales link heartburn to a head full of hair, but whether that is true or not doesn't matter. What matters is relief! While most women swear by Tums, remember that they are filled with synthetic sugars, dyes and fillers – so order yourself some papaya enzymes instead! You'll thank me later.

Heartburn is One of the most common issues many women experience during pregnancy. What can you do to help? Your chiropractor may be able to provide relief, you probably have an underlying yeast and candida issue in your gut. So, you will have to watch what you eat to not flare up the yeast – look out for sugar, as yeast craves it.

Foods to limit:

* Coffee
* Chocolate
* Anything with Tomatoes
* Fried and fatty foods
* Sugars
* Dairy
* Carbohydrates

Foods to eat:
High alkalizing fruits and veggies. These include (but are not limited to):

* Apples
* Bananas
* Berries
* Dates
* Oranges
* Melons
* Beets
* Carrots
* Green Beans
* Mushrooms
* Peppers

You may find eating small meals or snacks throughout the day beneficial instead of large meals. You will for sure want to do this towards the end of your pregnancy as the baby is taking up more room.

Probiotics and **digestive enzymes** are amazing to help with heartburn! The probiotics will help to repopulate the gut with the good bacteria and fight yeast, while the digestive enzymes will help to break down foods and make them more easily digestible as well and helping to absorb more vitamins and minerals.

Papaya Enzyme is helpful to digest foods and can help with heartburn during pregnancy. You can either eat papaya itself or take it in a supplement as you are eating.

Vitamin D and **Magnesium** can help as well. (You knew Vitamin D would be listed, right?) You should also know that heartburn medication reduces calcium and magnesium. So, be careful! (112)

Lemon water helps to not only alkalize the body, but also helps to combat yeast and candida.

Coconut oil is great to not only great to cook in, but also to eat by itself. You will want to consume 2 tablespoons per day. One in the morning and one at night before bed.

As a chiropractor, I like to work on the cardiac sphincter. This is where the esophagus and the stomach meet. It is located right below the breastbone or xyphoid process. By using 2 fingers on both of your hands, you can push inward ½ to 1 inch and scoop downward towards your feet. Hold for 30 seconds to one minute. This should help stop heartburn from occurring. You can do this as often as you need to. After meals and at night are the best.

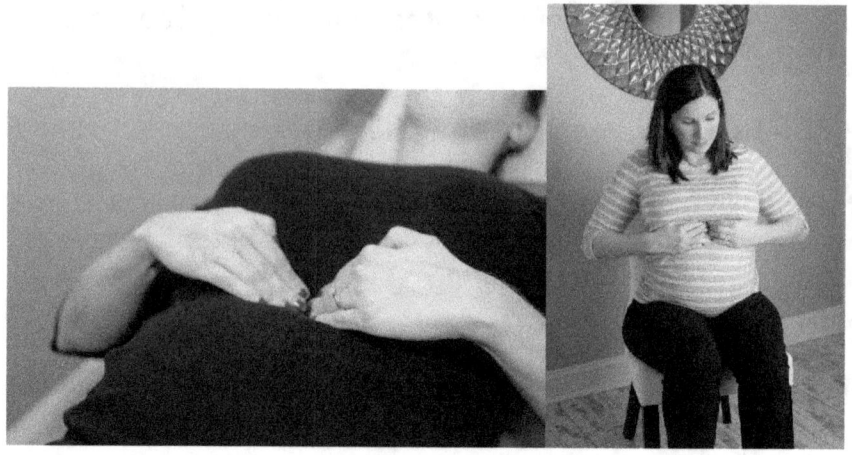

I also am a huge fan of **aloe juice**. This will help calm heartburn down. 4 oz in the morning and 4 ounces at night before you go to sleep will help with feeling better. I suggest you get something flavored. There will be some sugar as the flavoring, but regular aloe is very bitter and if you are already not feeling well, it may be hard to ingest. I feel the benefits outweigh the sugar in this case.

I have some pregnant moms feel better with **Apple Cider Vinegar**. 1-2 ounces throughout the day can help. Some add it to smoothies or some just drink it as a shot. You will have to test and try to find a way that works for you.

Adding 1-2 teaspoons of **baking soda** to a glass of water after meals can help with reducing acid. You may want to do this after eating some food as some women complain of an upset your stomach otherwise.

Adding **Ginger** to foods is helpful as well when dealing with the gut. It protects the lining of the stomach with its anti-inflammatory and anti-bacterial properties. This means it can help control a bacteria called helicobactor pylori or H. pylori from growing. These bacteria have been known to eat away at the lining of the stomach and cause ulcers. Some experience reflux/heartburn. The ginger can help with keeping it at bay.

Essential oils to help are: *peppermint, ginger, lemon, fennel.* Some companies have their own blend for digestion. I use the blends in my office all the time for constipation and gut issues. I use 4-5 drops in coconut and rub over the cardiac sphincter in this case.

This is not a complete list and you will have to see what works for you.

Low Back Pain and Sciatica

At some point during your pregnancy, you may experience some low back pain or sciatica. Sciatica can be experienced many different ways. Some will feel an electrical shock into the buttock or to the knee or foot and typically on one side, but I have had some moms have it in both legs. The shooting can be in the front or back of the leg. I have moms says they feel a burning or tingling in legs. Some moms complain of numbness in thighs. The sciatic nerve is very large and can be irritated by tight muscles, pelvis and sacrum misalignment, or due to the baby being in a sub-optimal position. Poor posture due to center of gravity being shifted may also be playing a role in your pain.

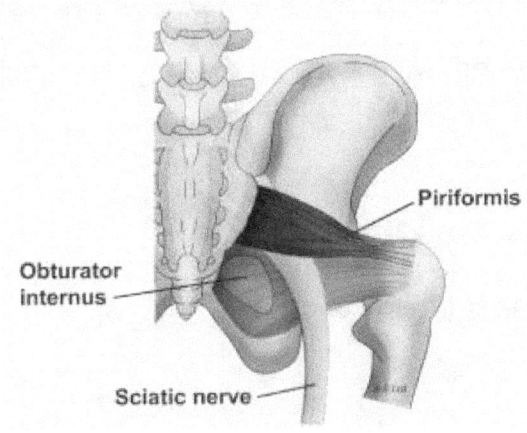

Many of my mom's to be are told this is all part of pregnancy and they just have to get through it. While the pain may last throughout pregnancy, there are ways to help manage low back pain and sciatica during pregnancy.

Apply Ice and _not heat_. Adding heat to an already inflamed muscle and nerve may feel good, but it can make the pain worse and increase the inflammation. So, ice is the best option to calm the muscle down and get rid of the swelling.

A trip to the **prenatal chiropractor** will help with aligning the maternal pelvis to help relieve your pain in a safe and non-invasive manner. Like I had said before, try to find a chiropractor trained in the Webster Technique as they are specialized in prenatal chiropractic care. (113)

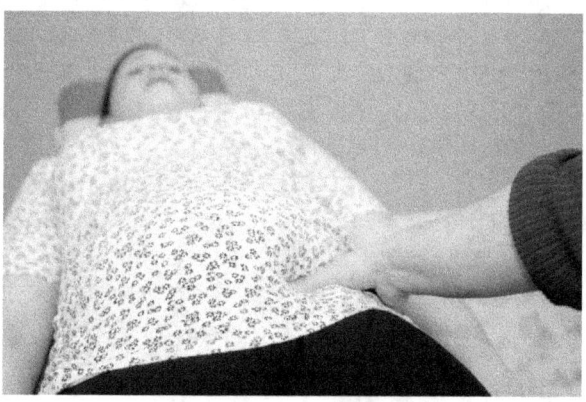

You should be enjoying your pregnancy and back pain does not have to define your pregnancy.

Did You Know?

Chiropractic care is more effective in treating low back pain than with standard medical care.
(114)(115)

Regular adjustments throughout pregnancy will not only help with pain, but they will aid in:
- Better sleep
- Easier movement
- Less round and broad ligament pain (groin pain)
- More efficient exercising
- Allowing baby to move into a better position
- Shortening labor time
- Helping to boost the immune system

Prenatal Massage also helps to reduce tension in the muscles to decrease low back pain. A good massage can increase oxygen to the body and improve circulation. It helps to drain lymph nodes which reduces swelling and boosts your immune system. According to the *American Pregnancy Association*, not only does prenatal massage help physically, but also mentally, as well as helping to regulate hormones. (116)

Just like chiropractors, not all massage therapist are specialized in prenatal massage. So, it is important to find a masseuse you are comfortable with and is knowledgeable about the body during pregnancy. In my office, we typically do not see pregnant women until at least week 15 or possibly longer depending on prenatal history. If moms to be have been under my care to oversee their health and wellness in pregnancy, I will recommend massage on case by case basis. If no complications, I may OK the massage ahead of time. It is always good to consult with your OBGYN or midwife first before you receive a massage as a precaution.

Vitamin D is also wonderful in helping to control low back pain and chronic pain in general. (117)(118)
I will remind you again, please make sure your health practitioner has checked your Vitamin D levels. A simple blood test can tell you where your levels are. You should be supplementing with a daily dose unless you happen to live in

a very sunny area where you are getting sunlight in peak hours between 12-2PM for 10 to 15 minutes per day. According the Vitamin D Council, pregnant and nursing mothers should be taking 4-6,000 IU's of vitamin D per day with upper end 10,000. (119)

I like to recommend liquid over capsules or tablets. I have done lab testing and have found the liquid far more superior in absorption than pill form. There are many great brands. Xymogen, DaVinci, or Klaire to name a few. I also like to have my mom's take their Vitamin D at night as it can help you sleep better too.

Prenatal Yoga can help with your back pain. Yoga helps to improve posture and gives you the ability to relax throughout pregnancy. The breathing techniques you will learn can also be used during labor. The increased oxygen to the body will help improve circulation not only to you, but your baby as well. This will also allow you to in turn in your sleep easier and have a clearer mind. Getting more sleep can help rejuvenate the body and help with easing your back pain. (120) A few of my favorite poses are the cat and cow (pelvic rocks!) as well as child's pose.

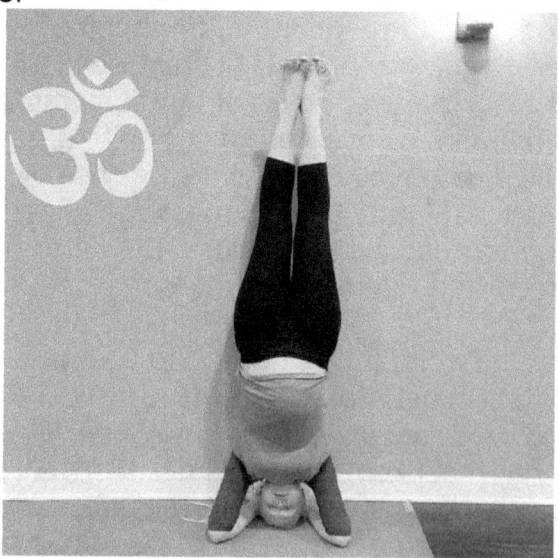

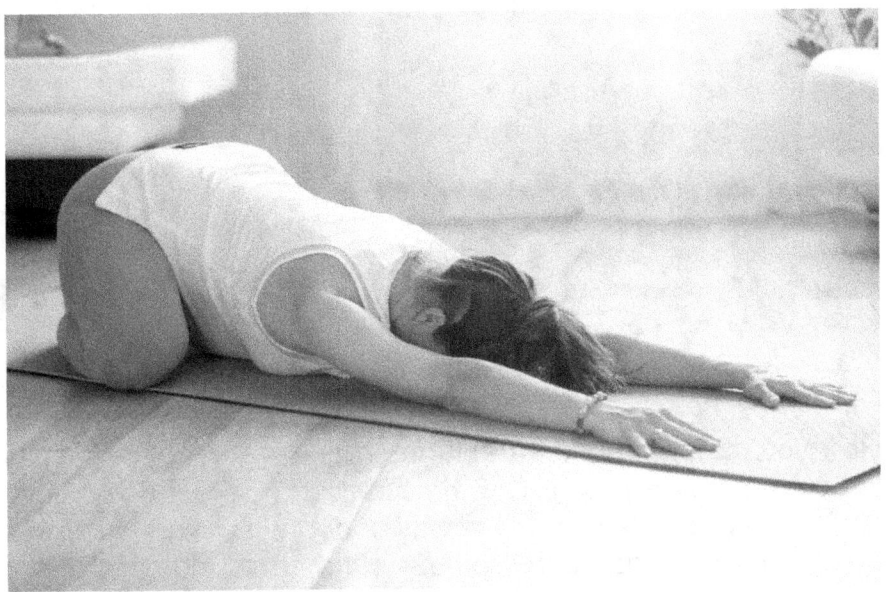

Carpal Tunnel Syndrome (CTS)

There is nothing fun about having carpal tunnel. Waking up in the middle of the night with your hands asleep can be scary. Some women have shooting pains while other women can't hold on to a coffee mug or take a lid off a jar. All of these are, unfortunately, common during pregnancy. CTS is not always easy to treat. What works for one mom, may not work for another. We have to try to manage the CTS the best we can. The good news is it usually goes away within a few short days of having your baby.

CTS is inflammation of the median nerve. This nerve actually come from the neck which we term the Brachial Plexus. As you can see, it is very complex and goes under many muscles(pectoralis) and goes all the way to the hand.

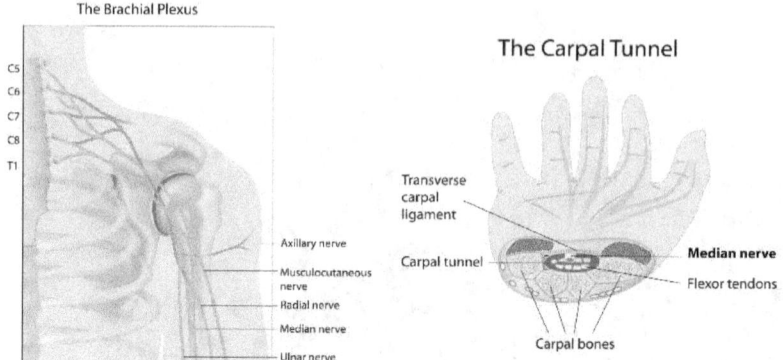

How you can manage carpal tunnel:
- Improving posture of the head and neck. Stretching the pec muscles on the wall or doorway. This will allow more blood and nerve flow to the arms and hands.
- Icing the neck and shoulders can help with reducing the swelling and tension in the muscles. Also keeping the house cooler in the summer will help as well. Make sure you are drinking plenty of water as well!

Once again, chiropractic care can help with aligning the body and help to take the pressure off the median nerve. It will also help to loosen up the muscles and help to restore nerve flow back to the hands to calm the carpal tunnel down.
Some people find hand splits to wear at night helpful with carpal tunnel and allow moms to be get some sleep.

Many pregnant women have found supplementing with B complex to be helpful, especially B6, in aiding to calm the nerve pain down. Others have found magnesium work wonders.

Headaches

Headaches during pregnancy can be frustrating because there's not much you can do for them. The headaches can come from many different things:
- Dehydration

- Hormones
- Lack of sleep
- Poor posture
- A combination of all of the above

Many doctors will prescribe Tylenol, but you have already learned why that is not a good decision.

Chiropractic care is one of the safest ways to help with headaches during pregnancy. It is not invasive. It is drug free, and it helps to align the body to function better. This allows the headaches to improve over time. (121)

Headaches can also come from low vitamin D. (This shouldn't surprise you!) Sometimes low magnesium. And sometimes they can come from B vitamins, whether your levels are too high or too low. Again, having your vitamin levels checked is important!

Peppermint oil is an easy alternative to help with headaches. You can add a drop to your wrists, behind your ears, or you can always add a few drops to water and diffuse in the room.

Make sure you are breathing plenty of oxygen. Because of our stressed out society we tend to 'shallow breathe.' Taking in deep breaths -in through the nose and out the mouth- can help increase your oxygen supply to you and your baby. You will want to do this throughout the day or any time you feel a headache coming on.

You will want to make sure you are also eating enough throughout the day. The added calories needed throughout the pregnancy need to be met. It's great to have snacks around. This will also help to regulate blood sugars so you won't have highs and lows throughout the day.

Other Common Pregnancy Ailments

Acne: All of the hormones running through your body are to blame for acne. Make sure to wash your face daily with a natural product and keep the skin properly moisturized. Adjusting your diet and eliminating dairy and gluten may also help.

Anxiety and Fears: This may just come with the pregnancy territory and of course depends on each woman's individual personality. Pregnancy is full of unknowns, parenthood is full of unknowns. Anxiety is normal, but if you feel as though it is hindering your life or taking over your thoughts, speak to your birth team as soon as possible.

Body Hair: You may become harrier while pregnant- hair on your breasts, abdomen, and face may show up out of nowhere. But on the flip side, you may notice that your arm and leg hair growth radically slows down. The hormones are responsible and again, you may want to have a blood panel done to know if you are deficient in any vitamins or minerals.

Braxton hicks: These vary from woman to woman and pregnancy to pregnancy. Consider them exercises for the uterus. They are very valuable and should not scare you. Braxton Hicks prepare the uterus for labor. Most women describe them as a tightening of the abdomen. They may make you catch your breath at times. If they happen frequently, try to lower your stress level, lay down, take a bath, and relax. If they continue at more than 6 an hour, contact your birth team.

Change in eye sight: This is not as common as other ailments, but it is classified as normal. Work with your eye doctor closely, as you may need a new prescription, but remember that it may return to normal once baby arrives.

Cold Symptoms: This may seem to be an odd pregnancy symptom, but it is quite common. Most women just don't link it to pregnancy. There is excess mucus that is present and can cause sinus pressure, sore throat, and everything else "cold-like." It should level out, but talk to your birth team if not.

Constipation: Your prenatal vitamin can be to blame, or just the pregnancy. Try to increase your fiber intake and start taking magnesium. Exercise should also help the bowels function better.

Cramps/Abdominal Pain: Unless the cramping intensifies or bleeding occurs, cramping typically means the uterus is growing. This is the number one complaint and scare throughout pregnancy. If you are scared, please visit your birth team. They will be there to reassure you.

Decreased hunger: As your uterus grows, there is less room to fill the stomach. You will need to eat smaller meals more frequently to keep satisfied, but it is common to lose interest in food due to nausea or food smells. If you fall into this category, really try to keep healthy protein snacks on hand to eat throughout the day.

Diarrhea: The body may not enjoy the same foods while pregnant. You may find dairy or gluten may trigger this ailment. Keep a food journal to find the root cause of your diarrhea.

Exhaustion: First and third trimester exhaustion is well known, but don't panic if the energy doesn't return in the second trimester. Increasing your iron intake can help tremendously. (122)

Freezing: The internal thermostat may shift the opposite way and turn you into an ice chest! Sometimes the seasons come into play with this temperature shift. Layering your clothes, keeping a sweater nearby, and wearing warm socks may help. Don't deny yourself a nice warm bath!

Gas: This is one of the more embarrassing side effects of pregnancy. The progesterone in your body plays a role in this excessive gas. Progesterone slows the digestive process, causing the horrible bloated feeling and gas to occur. Keep a food journal to figure out the foods that may be triggering the gas and eat smaller more frequent meals.

Hair Loss: You may have heard that your hair starts falling out after your baby is born, but for some women, it happens while pregnant. This can be a bit frightening, but it should not be harmful. There is a chance that your thyroid is acting out and signaling something deeper than pregnancy causing this hair loss though. Having your thyroid checked through a blood work panel is a good idea. (123) (124)

Hemorrhoids: These can develop internally or externally in the rectum or anus. They can burn or itch. Hemorrhoids are basically varicose veins of the rectum, and with increased blood flow during pregnancy they can develop easily. You may notice blood around your stool or when you wipe, or you may experience an uncomfortable pressure in your rectum. Add more fiber into your diet to help ease the discomfort of going to the restroom. Witch hazel and warm sitz baths are known to help with hemorrhoids. Some, moms to be find coconut oil not only in their diet, but externally can help with going to the bathroom easier. Aloe Vera gel can help as well.

Increased hunger: You are growing a human. This takes energy. Energy is fueled by what we put into our body. Make smart food choices. Increase your protein intake to stay fuller longer.

Increase sex drive: Thank you blood flow! As long as you have a willing partner, pregnancy can be a very orgasmic time. Work with your belly and comfort zones and enjoy sex. Sex is a wonderful form of exercise and provides many benefits emotionally and physically for you. Semen has natural "antibiotics" that line the cervix to prevent infection – it also helps soften the cervix to help prepare for labor.

Increased urination: This is due to constant pressure on your bladder from the growing uterus. So anytime there is ANY urine in the bladder, you feel as though you need to pee immediately. It may be worse if baby is sitting very low.

Insomnia: You can take a lavender bath by placing a drop of lavender oil in your bath water - on your pillow at night. Plug in a sleep machine, and exercise regularly to help the body prepare for sleep. Herbs to take according to Euphoric Herbals are Oat Straw and Skull Cap. I also like to recommend you take your Vitamin D at night as that can help you sleep as well. Magnesium and Epsom salt baths will help insomnia. Mediation to help lower cortisol and slow down the mind. Also, put away the phone and tablets as they can overstimulate the brain and not let you sleep.

Itchy Skin: While stretching and growing, the skin may become itchy. This can be a sign of stretch marks or a pregnancy rash, or it can just be a common annoyance. Keep the skin moisturized daily.

Knee pain: You may experience pain in your knees from standing or walking for long periods. Your feet become heavier in pregnancy and exert a lot more pressure on your muscles and joints. Make sure to prop your feet up to take the weight off, and wear a knee brace if it helps. Your chiropractor can also play a role in reliving some of the pain. Although limiting excess weight gain may be the best solution. If the pain persists, try a topical arnica rub and alternate between hot and cold compresses. Epsom salt baths to help with the swelling.

Leg and Foot Cramps: Many women suffer from daily or nightly leg or foot cramps. These can bring tears to your eyes and keep you from sleeping. Stretching, exercise, staying hydrated, and using magnesium (supplements or topically) will help with these cramps. Potassium is also great with helping cramps. Bananas or supplementation. Epsom salt baths also help with cramping. (128)

Mood Swings: You may experience tears, anger, and joy within a 45 second window of time. This is completely normal. Make sure you are eating regularly to keep you blood sugar levels within normal. However, if the feelings of sadness are overwhelming contact your birth team to talk.

Pregnancy Brain: This turns into "Mommy Brain" once baby arrives. Science acknowledges this – and short of slowing down and trying to focus on one task at a time, there's not much you can do. (126)

Metal Mouth: That metallic taste is not in your head. The taste buds can change during pregnancy – or your salivary glands are under producing. Eat saliva producing, juicy foods and brush your tongue regularly. Lemon water. You may also want to check you iron levels as the could be too high or too low.

Morning Sickness (All Day, Evening, or Night Nausea): All forms of nausea are normal throughout pregnancy. While most women see it lesson in the second trimester, others experience it up until their babies are born. Make sure that you are well hydrated and eating small meals often. Taking B-6, zinc, and increasing B-complex vitamins and iron intake tend to help with queasiness. According to Cindy Collins owner or Euphoric Herbals ginger and peppermint tea can help with nausea, as well as Red raspberry tea. Ginger gum have also been known to help.

Overheating: With blood flow increasing throughout pregnancy, you are going to feel a shift in your natural thermostat. You may become very warm and struggle with cooling down. Stay comfortable with cool showers and lukewarm baths frequently; sleep with a fan, wear light clothing, and stay hydrated.

Pigmentation: Change in the color of the skin can occur. Dark circles, discoloration, and extremely chapped lips can all show up one morning. Aloe Vero pulp may help, or lemon dipped in turmeric rubbed on the areas. Keeping up on Vitamin D will help too.

Poor bladder control: You've read about doing kegel exercises. If you are experiencing bladder issues, you may want to increase you kegeling.

Prenatal Depression: Everyone has heard of post-partum depression, but becoming depressed while pregnant can also occur. It needs to be taken very seriously. Feelings of sadness may be common, but if you are feeling extremely sad, anxious, or depressed, please contact your birth team immediately for help. (125)

PUPP rash: A burning and itching unlike anything you can imagine. This rash is no joke! The most natural way to sooth this is by rubbing a banana peel over the rash. You can try oatmeal baths with backing soda.

Sensitive breasts: Your breasts will change and grow right along with your uterus. They are preparing to make colostrum and then milk for the baby. Warm or cold compresses may help.

Shortness of Breath: an increase in pregnancy hormones (progesterone) stimulate your brain to tell your lungs that they need to take in more air. The growing uterus adds pressure to the diaphragm, making it hard to take the deep breaths your body is craving. A chiropractor may help with correcting your posture, which can make getting air easier.

Spotting: Spotting throughout early pregnancy is very common, but very worrisome as well. There are several reasons this can occur and still lead to a very healthy pregnancy and delivery. Spotting after sex is also very common. However, if you are cramping and spotting, there is a higher cause to worry. Call your birth team to be seen. (127)

Stretch marks: Most stretch marks are linked to genetics. You can use a cocoa butter lotion or other natural products, and they may help, but if it's in your DNA to leave marks as you grow, it may be out of your hands. Keep in mind that they should fade after pregnancy.

Swelling: This is dangerous territory. It is normal to complain about slight swelling, but if you swell suddenly or overnight, you need to have your blood pressure taken immediately, as this is a warning sign to pre-eclampsia. Contact your birth team if your swelling is concerning you at all. Rest, use ice, take a bath, and look at your diet to help reduce swelling.

Varicose Veins: Enlarged, bluish bulging vessels that have been stretched and weakened may appear. Blood accumulates here and results in cramping, aching and heaviness. Avoid standing or sitting for long periods and wear lose fitting garments. (129)

Vivid Dreams: Ranging from orgasmic to terrifying, all of these new hormones can mess with your dreams. Don't feel guilty or upset by these, as they have no significant meaning – THANK GOODNESS, but if they have you extremely worried, you can talk to your midwife.

Vomiting: A step further than morning sickness, vomiting can be debilitating to some women. Depending on the severity, your birth team may decide that medication is needed. Although, that should be the last resort. To help, avoid triggers such as certain smells or textured foods that cause you to vomit.

Weight gain: Weight gain can cause pains and problems, discomforts and emotions. Your weight will change while pregnant. By exercising and eating a healthy, well-balanced diet of whole, real foods, you will minimize the complaints that come along with weight gain.

Yeast Infections: High amounts of estrogen secreted during pregnancy can cause the vagina to remain moist. This makes it easy for yeast to grow. Estrogen also speeds the growth and enables the yeast to stick to the vagina. Air out the area often and cut out sugar from your diet. Also, don't forget the coconut oil and lemon in your water.

Zero sex drive: And then there are those who have absolutely no interest in having sex while pregnant. I tend to find women on one side of the spectrum or the other. Keep an open communication with your partner if you feel this way. It can cause tension and unwanted arguing if you keep your feelings to yourself. It is common to begin a pregnancy in this stage and by half-way through have an increased sex drive again.

Chapter 10
Food Cravings and Their Meanings

Pregnancy cravings are real, and our society has categorized pregnancy as a period of time in which women should eat whatever they want, in whatever portion size they crave. This is just absurd and dangerous to the health of the mother and baby.

Food cravings are a sign that **the body is lacking something.** Many women crave strange food combinations, leading to giggles and very odd snacks, but the body is searching for something. The body is asking to be fed the right nutrients.

I want to be clear that there is a difference between enjoying a food and *craving* a food. I am talking about real cravings in this chapter.

You know you need to be taking a high quality prenatal vitamin, possibly other supplements to meet your body's needs as well; but what you don't realize that the body still may be begging you for something else.

Don't get me wrong, there is a time and place to give in to a craving. Just understand that the body desires something more.

Did You Know?

Studies are showing that salty cravings do not increase the risk of gestational diabetes, but the sweet cravings do. Not only does craving sweets increase the risk of gestational diabetes, but it also increases the chances of excess weight gain and obesity with the mother and baby.

(130)(131)

<u>Note: Don't forget to eat organic for best nutritional benefits</u>.

Sweets

Chocolate

It's not surprising that chocolate comes up as the most common craving; it works on the endorphins and makes a person feel good! Chocolate's phenylethylamine can make you feel relaxed, not to forget that it is loaded with magnesium.

What your body really wants is **Magnesium.** Magnesium is a mineral that is vital to several functions of the body, including relaxing blood vessels and providing us with energy.

Did You Know?

The hippocampus is a part of the brain that is connected with emotion. It has a high concentration of magnesium (132), which may be the link between emotions and a sweet tooth!

Meet the craving:

- Dark chocolate
- Nuts and seeds
- Bananas and Avocados

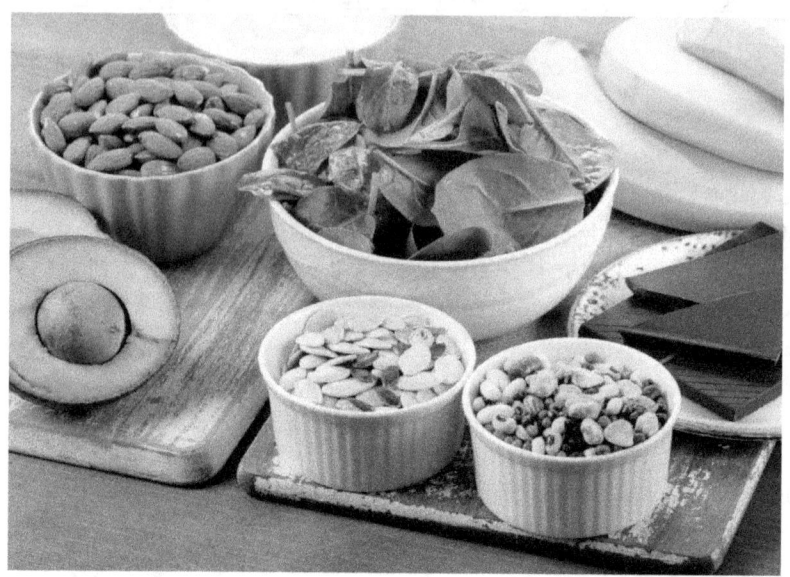

You may also meet the craving by taking a nice bath with magnesium flakes, or even a foot soak with magnesium. A magnesium lotion or oil can be used topically to help the body meet its magnesium needs as well.

Sugar

One craving that is hard to kick is a sugar craving. We are all basically addicted to it, so there is no question as to why we crave it. Most sweets offer nothing in the way of nutrition.

What your body really wants is **Chromium, Carbon, Sulfur, Tryptophan, Phosphorus and Glucose.**

Your body does need some natural sugar to make it through the day and keep your blood glucose levels where they should be; and abstaining from all forms of sugar may not be a sustainable goal for you. Chromium has been linked to glucose metabolism, and helps to balance blood sugar levels. (133)

Meet the craving:
- Fruit
- Vegetables
- Sweet Potatoes

Carbon is found in fresh fruits. (134)

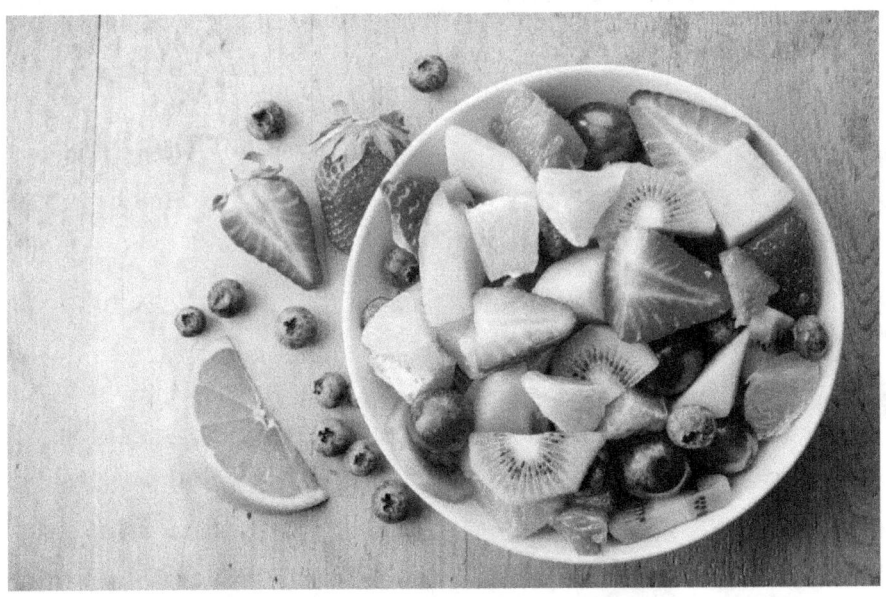

Bread

Bread turns to sugar in the body. Yes, the same sugar that I just mentioned that is addicting. There is even more to be concerned with here, though. Our country's grains are being sprayed with pesticides (like RoundUp) causing many gut issues and other complications within the body (and fetus).

What your body really wants is **Amino Acids and Nitrogen**. Amino acids are produced by consuming protein. Your baby is receiving amino acids at a rapid rate through the placenta, so eating high-quality protein often is extremely important. (135)

Meet the craving:

- Plant and animal proteins are composed of more than 20 individual amino acids.
- Nuts and Seeds.
- Meat.
- Dark, Leafy Greens.

Salty Foods

Not all salts are the same. Most snacks and processed foods are made with low-quality salt.

What your body really wants is **Sodium.**

Table salt or the industrial-grade salt used in snacks should be avoided. This form of salt leads to fluid retention, which can cause weight gain and an increase in your blood pressure. However, sodium is important to a healthy diet. (137)

Meet the craving: Go with Himalayan pink salt or sea salt as natural sources of sodium.

Coffee

It's not coffee that is bad, it is the caffeine and any added sugar you mix in that causes your cravings.

What your body really wants is **Energy.**

Coffee may boost your energy, but it is not a long term fix.

Meet the craving:
- Protein
- Exercise

Fried or Oily Foods

It's hard to say no to fried chicken. I understand, but if you are eating it due to cravings consider the reason.

What your body really wants is **Healthy Fats and Calcium.**

Healthy fats will help you feel full. Craving oily foods can be a sign of calcium deficiency.

Meet the craving:
- Avocados
- Almonds

- Cashews
- Olive Oil
- Broccoli
- Asparagus

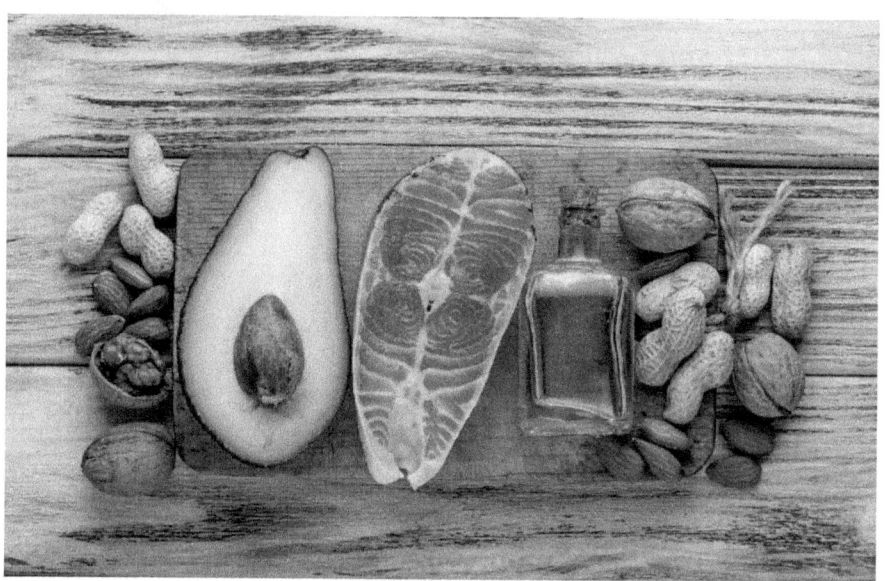

Protein

This craving is self-explanatory, but VERY important, especially during pregnancy!

What your body really wants is **Protein.**

Protein is a key ingredient to a healthy pregnancy.

Meet the craving:

Even though you may be craving fatty protein sources, you want to make sure that you are eating high-quality, grass-fed, hormone-free, lean protein as much as possible. Small meals and snacks throughout the day should level out your craving.

If you do not eat meat:

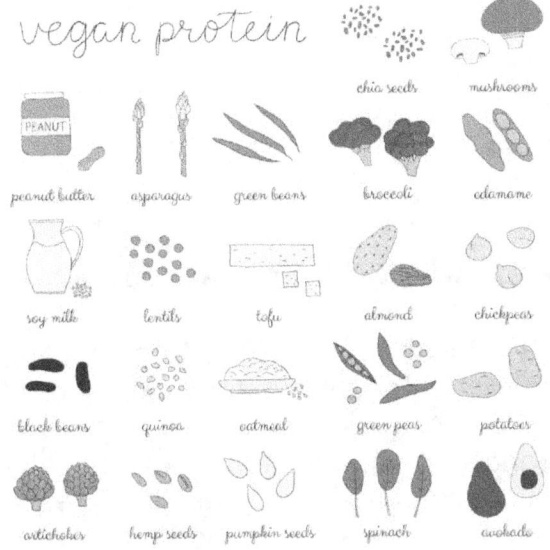

vegan protein

chia seeds • mushrooms

peanut butter • asparagus • green beans • broccoli • edamame

soy milk • lentils • tofu • almond • chickpeas

black beans • quinoa • oatmeal • green peas • potatoes

artichokes • hemp seeds • pumpkin seeds • spinach • avocado

No Cravings, but a Loss in Appetite

Lack of cravings is actually a craving. Confused? I'll bet. Hear me out. If you are not craving anything at all, as in food means just about nothing to you other than a quick meal, it could be that you're not getting enough vitamins and minerals.

What your body really wants is **Zinc.** Zinc affects your taste buds and could be behind you lack of enthusiasm over food.

Meet the (lack of) craving:

Eat a variety of proteins, fruits, and vegetables to cover all of your nutritional bases. You should feel your appetite return after a few days of healthy eating. If your lack of appetite is persistent check with your doctor to uncover potential causes. Specific foods that contain zinc:

- Spinach
- Carrots
- Lentils
- Shrimp
- Sunflower Seeds

A Proposed Model of Craving Etiology

"Craving is hypothesized to be due to competing approach-avoidance conflicts brought about by exposure to foods that are perceived as being simultaneously appealing (due to an innate preference for high-calorie, sweet, and fatty foods) and forbidden (due to cultural norms prescribing restrained intake and a thin figure). While most individuals are thought to attempt to resolve the resulting ambivalence in favor of abstinence (represented by the solid lines), pregnancy is hypothesized to be a culturally sanctioned permissive factor, allowing women to circumvent their usual conflicting response and efforts to restrict intake and indulge in foods that they would otherwise avoid, resulting in increased intake and heightened risk for weight gain specifically during pregnancy (represented by the dashed lines)."

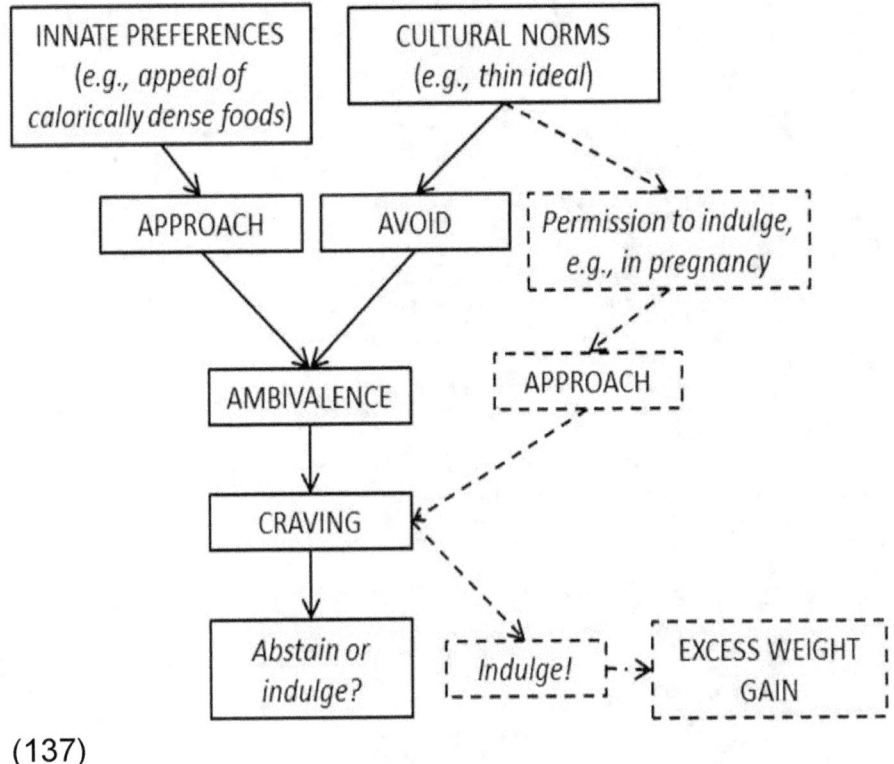

(137)

IF YOU CRAVE	YOU NEED	FOODS THAT SATISFY YOUR CRAVING
Chocolate	Magnesium	Raw nuts and seeds, legumes, fruits
Sweets	Chromium	Broccoli, grapes, cheese, dried beans
	Carbon	Fresh fruits
	Phosphorus	Fish, eggs, dairy, nuts, legumes
	Sulfur	Cranberries, horseradish, cruciferous vegetables, kale, cabbage
	Tryptophan	Cheese, lamb, raisins, sweet potato, spinach
Bread/toast	Nitrogen	High protein foods
Oily snacks, fatty foods	Calcium	Mustard and turnip greens, broccoli, kale, legumes, cheese, sesame
Coffee/tea	Phosphorous	Beef, liver, poultry, fish, eggs, dairy, nuts, legumes
	Sulfur	Egg yolks, red peppers, muscle protein, garlic, onion, cruciferous vegetables
	NaCl (salt)	Sea salt, apple cider vinegar
	Iron	Meat, fish and poultry, seaweed, greens, black cherries
Alcohol, Rec. Drugs	Protein	Meat, poultry, seafood, nuts
	Avenin	Steel Cut Oats
	Calcium	Mustard and turnip greens, broccoli, kale, legumes, cheese, sesame
	Glutamine	Supplement glutamine powder, raw cabbage juice
	Potassium	Sun-dried black olives, potato peel broth, seaweed, bitter greens
Chewing Ice	Iron	Meat, fish and poultry, seaweed, greens, black cherries
Burned Food	Carbon	Fresh fruits
Soda and Carbonation	Calcium	Mustard and turnip greens, kale, legumes, cheese, sesame
Salty Foods	Chloride	Raw goat milk, fish, unrefined sea salt
Acid Foods	Magnesium	Raw nuts and seeds, legumes, fruits
Preference for liquids rather than solids	Water	Flavor water with lemon or limes
Cool Drinks	Manganese	Walnuts, almonds, pecans, pineapple, blueberries
Menstrual Cravings	Zinc	Seafood, leafy veggies, root veggies
Overeating	Silicon	Nuts, seeds; avoid refined starches
	Tryptophan	Cheese, lamb, raisins, sweet potato, spinach
	Tyrosine	Vitamin C supplements, or orange, green, red fruits and veggies

1. Lectures, Cheryl M. Deroin, NMD, Southwest College of Naturopathic Medicine, Spring 2003 (healthy food recommendations)
2. Benard Jenson, PhD, The Chemistry of Man B. Jensen Publisher, 1983 (deficiencies linked to specific cravings and some food recommendations)

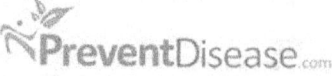

Chapter 11

The Benefit of Sex During Pregnancy and How to Increase Sex Drive

I have talked about what you should be putting in to your body, and the best ways to stay healthy, but now it's time to talk about something that most couples rarely discuss while pregnant: SEX.
It seems to be something that is never covered by doctors. It's never brought up during appointments, and too embarrassing to ask about, right?

WRONG.

Sex is what got you pregnant. It is natural. It is animalistic even. It is what our bodies are designed to do. So let's lose the embarrassment and start talking.

Sex During Pregnancy:

38% of women claim to have an increased libido while pregnant, and close to 50% of women admit that their pleasure during sex was immensely more intense than pre-pregnancy. (138)

If you can muster up even an inkling of wanting to have sex, I highly recommend it. The more frequently you do the deed, the more your body will crave it. (However, no means no – do not let anyone talk you into something you are not comfortable doing. Not even your partner.)
It is so easy to let pregnancy be your excuse to not have sex. The body is going through so much right now. You are gaining weight, changing shape, feeling hormonal, and just plain

different than before pregnancy. The sex drive may naturally crash, but I promise that sex can still be good.

The first thing you need to let go of is thinking that you can harm the baby. Having sex will *not* hurt the baby. You can potentially cause a little bit of bleeding with deep penetration (especially in the first trimester), but it's nothing to be scared of, no harm to the pregnancy is done at all.

Fortunately for everybody involved, except for in rare cases, sex is totally awesome for both you and your baby! Even while your sex drive will most definitely fluctuate throughout pregnancy, there will probably be some libido *highs.* At these points, GO FOR IT! Roll around in the sheets – swing from the chandelier! I bet your orgasm will be amazing. Something about those pregnancy hormones makes for over the top orgasms.

Sex Safety

Sex is perfectly safe throughout the entire pregnancy, up until the water breaks. Once the water breaks, nothing should be going "in," only a baby should be coming out! The uterus, along with the amniotic sac, will protect your baby. The thick mucus plug that seals the cervix also helps guard against infection. (If you have lost your mucus plug, don't fret, it regrows!) Just in case all of those protective measures aren't enough, the semen act as a natural antibiotic to prevent infection too! (139)

It's almost as if our bodies were designed it do this. Oh, wait... they are!

Note: Orgasms may cause mild uterine contractions (as can nipple stimulation), yet they are both temporary and harmless. You will not trigger labor *unless your baby is ready to be born.* Your midwife or doctor will tell you to abstain if there is medical reasoning.

Sex Truths and Benefits While Pregnant

Orgasm: The excess blood flow in pregnancy allows for a more sensitive and intense feeling during an orgasm.

Sex is Exercise: Sex assists your muscles to work strongly and effectively. It also gives your pelvic floor a nice workout. You know those kegels I have mentioned? Go ahead and practice them during sex too, your partner will barely be able to utter the words "Thank You."

Sex Lowers Blood Pressure: Regular sex during pregnancy, particularly in the second trimester, is effective in lowering systolic blood pressure. (Sex and orgasms produce progesterone, the hormone that relaxes blood vessels, decreasing blood pressure.) A lower blood pressure keeps preeclampsia away. (140)(141)

Maintains and Strengthens the Bond with Your Partner: A partnership that includes regular sexual intercourse, even throughout pregnancy, may be happier and feel closer than one that does not.

Boosts immune System: Sex is known to improve the immune system. Research suggests that the more sex a person has, the less sick days they experience. This is especially true for you, the pregnant women whose immune system is suppressed by the growing baby! Increased levels of IgA antibodies can help you ward off colds and fevers. (142)(143)

Improves the immunological relationship between you and your baby:

Semen contain HLA-G modulates, which suppress a pregnant woman's immune reactions to the baby she is growing. HLA-G is absorbed through the vagina after ejaculation. (It may also be absorbed through the stomach if you ingest it during foreplay.) (144)

Since the fetus is technically a foreign item within the mother's body, her immune system may become defensive during pregnancy. This battle can be dangerous to both the mother and the baby. HLA-G can help the mother's body accept the baby.

Estrogen produced during an orgasm aids in the baby's development and helps stimulate hormone production in the adrenal gland. It also teaches the uterus how to respond to oxytocin.

Pain Reduction: It has been found that genital stimulation increases women's pain thresholds, most likely due to the release of endorphins. Actually having sex produces high doses of oxytocin, which dramatically increases your pain tolerance. (145)

Lowers stress levels: Oxytocin can help alleviate anxiety and stress by reducing cortisol levels in the body, and it lowers blood pressure. *Prolactin* is also produced after an orgasm. It helps you feel relaxed and sleepy. (146)

Sex Prepares the Cervix for Labor: Semen contains prostaglandins which help soften and dilate the cervix, possibly speeding and easing labor. The oxytocin produced is the primary hormone responsible for contractions. Remember, that you are not at risk to cause preterm labor, but if your baby is ready to be born, then sex is can be a natural induction method. (147)

Increased Postpartum Recovery Speed: Sex and orgasms increase the strength of pelvic floor muscles. Strengthened pelvic floor muscles speed up muscle healing in the days and weeks following birth. This may reduce postpartum bleeding time, and help you feel better, faster. (148)

Sex decreases the chance of preterm labor: A study by the Guttmacher Institute shows that women who'd had sex during weeks 29-36 of pregnancy had a *lower* risk of pre-term delivery than women who'd abstained. Another study shows that frequent intercourse (more than once a week) during weeks 23-27 significantly reduced the risk of preterm labor. Seeing as how both studies show wonderful results, all the more reason to have frequent sex weeks 23 through birth. (149) (150) (151) (152)

Sex Lowers the Risk of Preeclampsia - Even oral sex during pregnancy has been shown to reduce the risk of preeclampsia. As you have read, research shows that intercourse lowers blood pressure. (153)

No Sexual Desires?

You are not alone; a lot of women are less sexually active in pregnancy. Reports show a decrease in desire, frequency and satisfaction during the first trimester, which then decreases the wanting of sex throughout the rest of pregnancy. But give it a go once you are feeling the slightest inkling of interest.

PART 2

A Breakdown of Pregnancy

The Natural Perspective of Growing a Baby

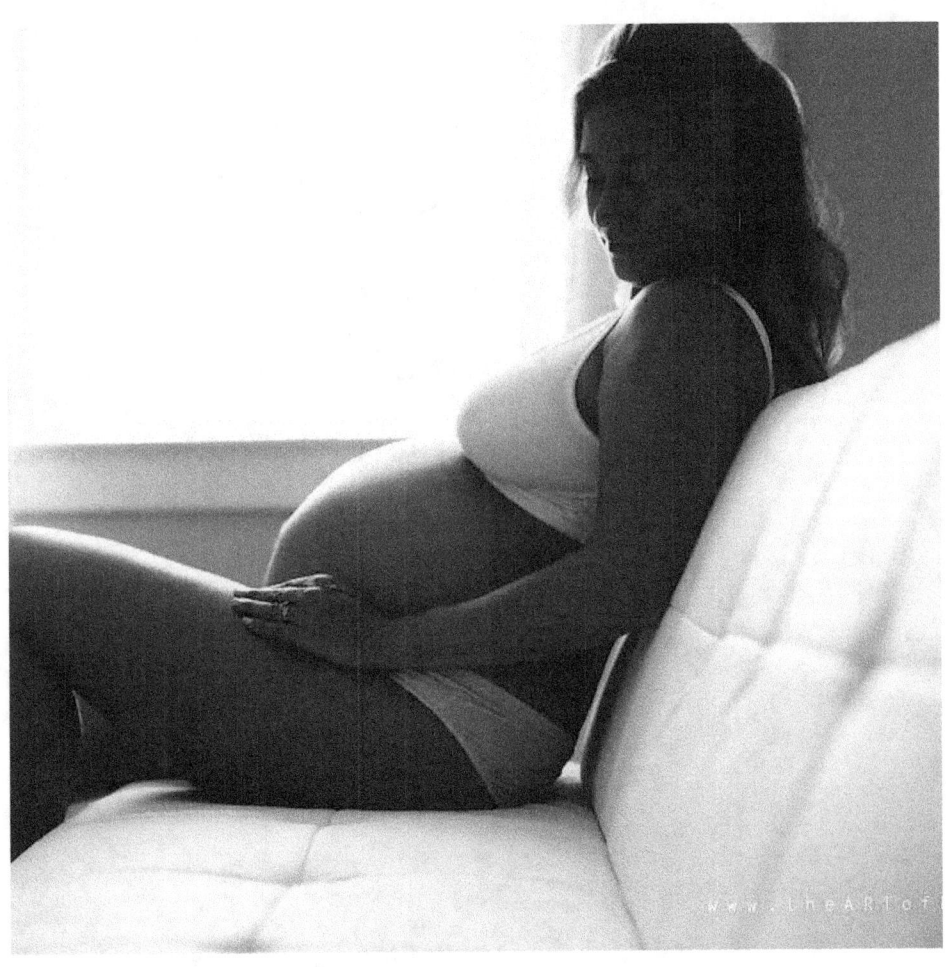

"Slow Down

Calm Down

Don't Worry

Don't Hurry

Trust The Process"

-Alexandra Stoddard

Chapter 12
The Amazing Uterus

Until puberty, you probably never thought about your uterus. Even then, you might have just hated it a few days each month. Hopefully, you have come a long way and understand how powerful and valuable this organ is.

A fun fact is that the vagina is actually INSIDE the body. What you see on the outside is the labia. The correct term for the entire area, "vulva" – NOT the vagina.

The uterus is a complex and muscular organ. It supports the bladder, bowel, pelvic bones and other surrounding organs. The uterus holds the bladder above the pubic bone and the bowel behind itself, keeping the two organs separate from each other.

Did You Know?

The #1 and #2 surgeries in our country are Cesarean Sections -the cutting of the uterus to remove a baby- and hysterectomies -the removal of the uterus, respectively. While a cesarean section leaves the uterus (mostly) intact, it permanently scars and possibly damages it.

Not only are we purposely removing and harming the uterus, but we are also causing damage in ways most people are very unaware. The uterus is penetrable and sensitive to chemicals and toxins. The problem is that our environment has become toxic; it is full of pollutants, products, and even foods filled with pesticides that are harming our bodies – including the uterus. If you don't think that is scary, then think about this: research is showing that hundreds of toxic chemicals are finding their way into the wombs of women. These chemicals are found within the amniotic fluid of pregnant mothers and are detectable within the blood of newborns – and the breastmilk of mothers. (154)

The Abilities of the Uterus

A healthy uterus increases to 1,000 times its original size during pregnancy. (155)

According to healing arts and holistic educator **Kara Maria Ananda,** the uterus has seven amazing abilities.

Sex

During sex, the uterus contracts to help the sperm in their journey to reach the egg. This contraction happens whether the cervix is open or closed, and throughout the woman's cycle – not just during ovulation. (156)

Strength

It has been argued that the uterus is the strongest muscle in the body by weight. As a woman who has given birth, I believe it to be true. There are layers of muscle tissue that construct this amazing organ and in labor, the uterus expels incredible pressure to push a baby out. Once you have experienced this, you too will believe the uterus to be the strongest muscle in the human body.

Flexibility

During pregnancy, a women's uterus grows and stretches until it reaches from the pelvic floor to the ribcage. Once birth occurs, it shrinks back to its original size. It is the ultimate rubber band.

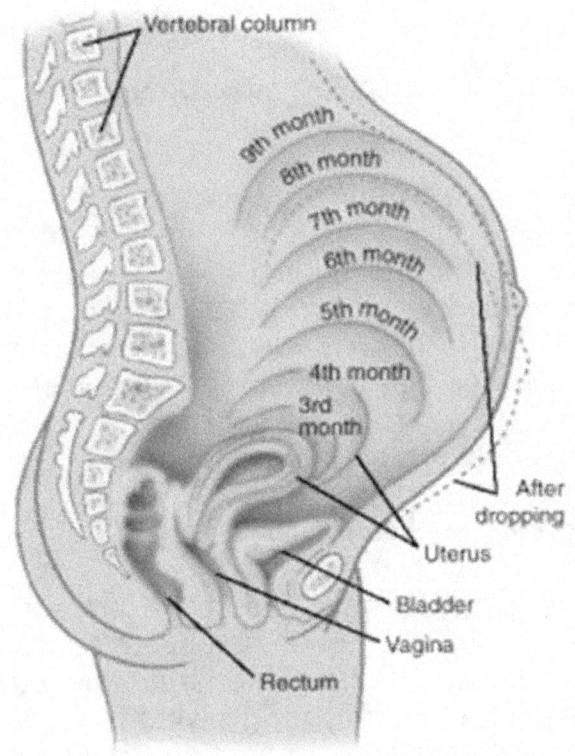

http://cancerlive.net/women-health/uterine-pregnancy/

Healing

Menstrual blood is rich in healing stem cells. This blood lines the uterus and awaits a fertilized egg to implant within it.

These stem cells are being researched to treat conditions such as stroke, heart disease, Parkinson's and diabetes. (157) According to neuroscience researchers from the University of South Florida, the stem cells found in menstrual blood have the ability to morph into various kinds of other cells. (158)(159)

Wouldn't it be amazing if we could find a greater use for menstrual blood?

Earth, Moon, Sun Cycles

Is it so hard to believe that our bodies are connected to the earth? The moon cycle is about 29 days and the average menstrual cycle is 28 days. With 13 moon cycles each year and the average age of first menstruation being about 13 years old (12.8 years is the average), it is easy to see that we are deeply rooted to our planet.

Growing a Foreign Organ

The uterus actually grows a new, foreign organ within itself: The placenta. Then this new organ *sustains a life.* As you will read in chapter 16, the placenta is absolutely amazing. It nourishes and feeds your growing fetus, and acts as the physical, life-support connection from you to your baby. It becomes even more amazing when you learn that the placenta acts as a sponge for nutrients but yet a barrier to the transferring of your blood to your baby. The placenta is the most unresearched organ, and there is still so much to learn about it.

Growing a Human

The uterus homes the entire area in which a tiny human is created and grown. From the release of an egg at ovulation, to the fertilization and implantation, to the growth of a placenta and multiplying cells until a fetus has formed. It grows in size to accommodate the fetus. It protects and nourishes. It is simply amazing.

Chapter 13
The First Trimester for Mom

When you first learn that you are pregnant, your body may have no noticeable external signs. This does not mean that nothing is changing. There is so much happening within you that is not visible to the naked eye.

The Conception

The first trimester begins on the first day of the last menstrual cycle. About two weeks from this date, the ovaries release a mature egg, and a sperm makes its way into this egg – fertilizing it - and it then imbeds into the uterine wall, implanting itself into the healthiest place possible. And now a pregnancy is officially underway.

Hormones

As the egg develops into a zygote, and further into an embryo, the mother's body *feels* the changes because of the hormonal shifts taking place.

As I have mentioned, HCG levels will double approximately every 48 hours from the moment of conception until about the 10th week of pregnancy. HCG is a hormone that is not present unless pregnancy occurs; therefore, the body will react to it until the hormone levels off. HCG circulates through the body and is eliminated through the urine. (This is the hormone that pregnancy tests are looking for to confirm conception.)

Days after Ovulation	Average hCG mIU/ml	Minimum-Maximum mIU/ml
14	48	17-119
15	59	17-147
16	95	33-223
17	132	17-429
18	292	70-758
19	303	111-514
20	522	135-1,690
21	1,061	324-4,130
22	1,287	185-3,279
23	2,034	506-4,660
24	2,637	540-10,000

Progesterone and estrogen are both increasing at this time, also playing a part in all pregnancy signs and symptoms for you. The placenta takes over producing these hormones around the 10th week of pregnancy. (160)

Estrogen helps the uterus grow, maintains the uterine lining, increases blood circulation, and stimulates the production of other hormones. It also causes the breasts to swell, along with many other pregnancy symptoms.

Progesterone is a vasoactive hormone, meaning that it can increase lower than normal blood pressure in pregnancy, (161) and it causes occasional dizziness, diarrhea, reflux, belching, nausea, vomiting, gas, and constipation.

Progesterone can also increase hair growth all over the body. It leads to the relaxation of the blood vessels throughout the entire body; so many of the first trimester pregnancy symptoms are tied to these hormones.

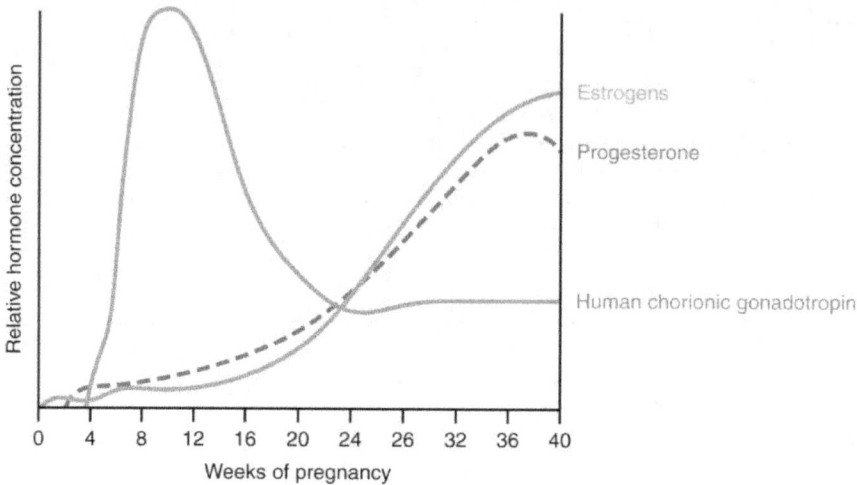

Early Signs and Positive Pregnancy Test

Many women say they feel pregnancy symptoms as early as 7-10 days past ovulation, but don't be alarmed if you don't. There may be implantation spotting that occurs around this time – or there may be no spotting. Inside the womb, the egg has split and cells have doubled numerous times, forming a zygote. Hormone levels are sky-rocketing and the your body may be feeling 'off.'

The earlier you take a HPT, the fainter the positive result will be. Each test brand requires a different amount of HCG hormone to be present in the urine, so waiting until the 4th week of pregnancy (2 weeks past ovulation) is highly recommended.

Scheduling an Appointment

It is important to begin interviewing your potential birth team early so you feel happy with your decision. While, the first appointment is not until about 10 weeks along, unless there is an appointment done to confirm pregnancy at an earlier date. The first appointment, depending on gestation, may include hearing the baby's heartbeat, which is always a monumental moment!

Body Changes

Bloating: It is quite typical to see bloating occur between weeks 4 and 10. This is due to the increase of hormones flowing through your body, but once the placenta takes over the production of hormones, the bloating should decrease. A true 'Baby Bump' is not really noticeable until further into the second trimester.

Swollen Breasts: Your breasts may be larger, perkier, and more tender during this stage of pregnancy.

First Trimester Possibilities

As you have read, there is quite the list of possible pregnancy complaints, and they may start as early as the 4th or 5th week of your pregnancy. A few of the earliest symptoms include:

Exhaustion: The body is working at exhausting levels to create the foundation of the healthiest pregnancy possible.

Spotting: Most women believe that a miscarriage is inevitable when spotting occurs, but that is not the case. 20-40% of pregnant women will experience bleeding during the first trimester, but continue on to have a healthy pregnancy. (162)

Cramping: Twinges and cramps are common and can be blamed on the round ligaments that are stretching and aiding in the growth of the uterus. Don't panic. Call your birth team if you are feeling scared.

Nausea/Vomiting: The increase in hormones circulating the body can cause nausea until the hormones level off. Typically by the end of the first trimester, nausea fades.

Food Aversions/Cravings: The body is on hyper-sensitive mode throughout weeks 4-12 of pregnancy. This includes smells, taste buds, and even food cravings. Remember what you have learned about food cravings.

Increased Heartrate: Cardiac volume increases by about 40 to 50% from the beginning to the end of the pregnancy. (163)

Weight Gain: While the average weight gain during the first trimester is about 5 pounds, some women actually lose weight because of morning sickness and food aversions.(164)

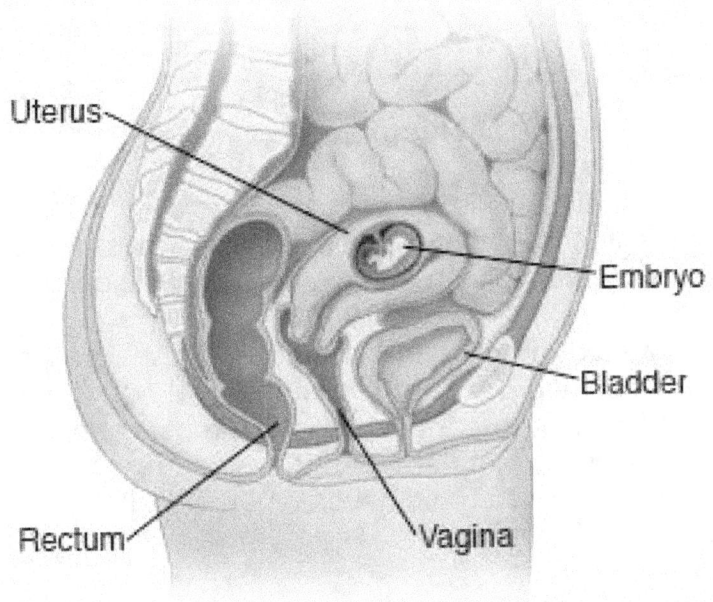

Uterus

Embryo

Bladder

Rectum

Vagina

The 'Safe' Zone

The end of the first trimester marks what most women label 'The Safe Zone.' If a heartbeat is heard, and measurements are in normal range, the chance of miscarriage drastically decreases. This is also the time that most people announce their pregnancies, as they have seen their midwife at least once and feel more comfortable in sharing the news.

Miscarriage occurs in about 20% of all pregnancies. There is not a direct cause that has been found, and typically, it cannot be prevented. Stressing about having a miscarriage is not productive, but living a healthy lifestyle is the best way to ensure you are doing everything to support a healthy pregnancy.

Things to Note

The first trimester is the most dramatic in terms of development for the baby. Smoking, drugs (over-the-counter even) can severely play a role in wrongful development.

In 2015, a study was released that shows the mother's gut flora can affect the development of the fetal brain as early as the first trimester of pregnancy. It is of utmost importance that a mother takes care of her diet and works on healing her gut to encourage positive brain development. (165)

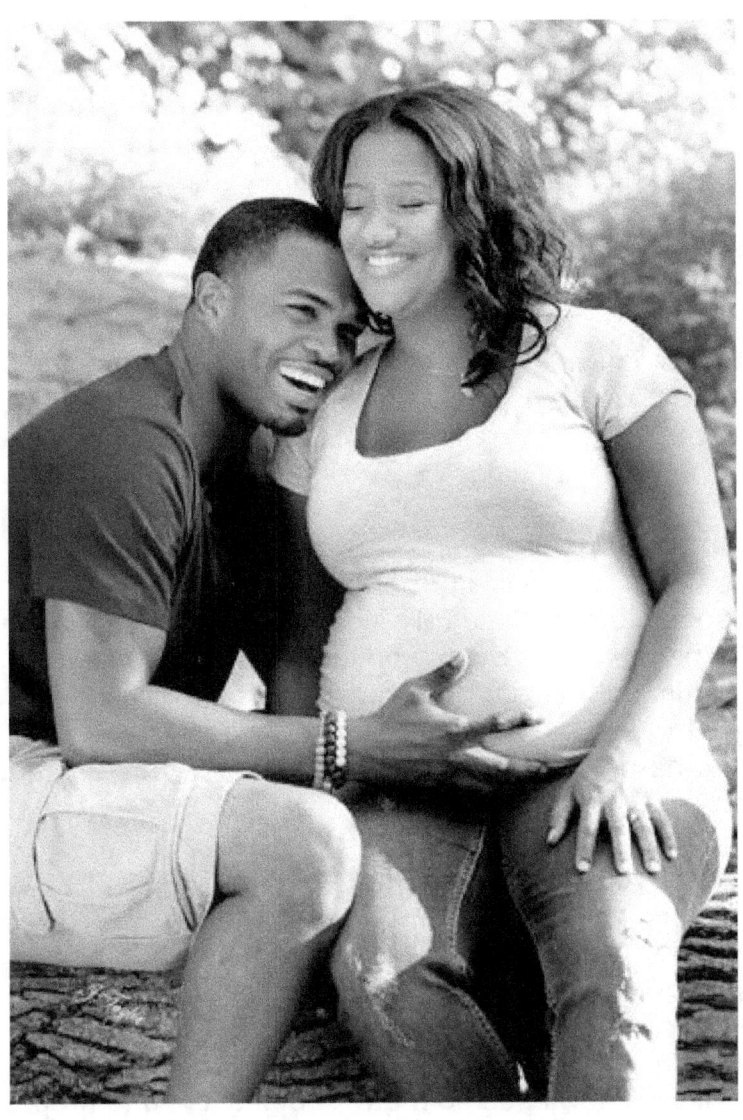

"The best thing a father can do for his children is to love their mother."
-John Wooden

Chapter 14
Tips for Partners During the First Trimester

This chapter is for the partners in the relationship.
Our society tends to only congratulate the mom, but the partner did partake in the making of this baby (in most cases). His life is changing too.

It's time to figure out your role in this whole pregnancy thing. It may be quite hard to commiserate with your partner because she looks no different, but yet is complaining about anything and everything.

There is so much happening below the surface for her though. Your partner is having hormone spikes that are sending her body up and down a wild rollercoaster. She has every right to take naps, as her body is working around the clock to grow this tiny implanted egg into a zygote, then an embryo, and finally into a fetus – all within the first trimester.
You will have to forgive the mood swings; they are nothing personal.

It is okay if you are terrified right about now. It's also okay to be over-the-moon excited. It's okay to have a whole mix of feelings going on. Know that you will be a great parent, and that you have a few months to figure this pregnancy and birth thing out.

As a chiropractor, I see so many couples trying to prepare for birth together. I highly recommend that you read 'Husband Coached Childbirth' or any other natural pregnancy and birth book. You want to understand what is going on throughout pregnancy and how to help support her as her partner.

I'm going to give you a brief overview of what to expect in the first trimester, and how you can be involved.

Month 1:

- Your partner will not see dramatic changes during the first month after conception.
- She may be abnormally, and what seems like excessively, tired. Make sure she gets rest, as it is very important early in pregnancy.
- Nausea may begin, and come in waves throughout the day. Remind her to eat small snacks often.
- Her breasts may become swollen and more tender. Reassure her that it is normal and that she looks beautiful.

Month 2:

- She may gain a small amount of weight or look a bit bloated.
- She will be exhausted. Her body is working very hard and she needs to rest.
- Your partner may have drastic mood swings. Her hormone levels are sky-rocketing and will cause her to be all over the place. She will go from happiness to tears over anything and everything.
- She may begin craving certain foods. Try to help her meet her cravings as healthily as possible. High-quality foods are very important, so think organic, unprocessed, non-gmo, free-range, and no antibiotics.

Month 3:

- Exhaustion hits an all-time high at this point, as the baby is growing into an actual fetus with working organs.
- She may either have an increased or decreased sex drive at this point. She may just be too tired to enjoy it. Be patient - this should not last, but supporting her through this stage is critical. Sex is completely safe, and even beneficial to pregnancy, but make sure your

partner is okay with any initiation you may want to make.

Things you can do in the first trimester:

Please know that your role during pregnancy is preparing you for your role as a parent. You are your partner's supporter during this time. *The best thing you can do is become involved and educated.*

1. Attend the first appointment: She is nervous; you are nervous, but together you will learn so much. You may even hear your baby's heartbeat!
2. Do the grocery shopping: Many women have severe food aversions and grocery stores can trigger them.
3. Do the cooking: Help ensure that she is eating a healthy diet, full of high quality protein and well-balanced sides.
4. Compliment her: Pregnancy is beautiful, even the beginning before the belly begins to swell. Help her embrace it by expressing how pretty she is each day.
5. Exercise with her: Make an evening walk together a new habit. Sign her up for prenatal yoga!
6. Stay connected: If intimacy is not enjoyable for your partner right now, find other ways to stay connected.
7. Destress: Try to keep all avoidable stress away from your partner. Stress can actually affect the development of the baby's brain in utero as early as the first trimester.
8. Take over finances: If possible, start saving money and live off one salary so you have the option of having a stay-at-home parent once baby arrives.
9. Talk about your emotions: Tell her how you feel. Share your fears and hopes, expectations and doubts. You will enjoy this pregnancy more if you feel emotionally invested.

Most partners worry about the future with children or want to put their partner in a bubble to protect them throughout pregnancy. My advice is this:

You cannot prevent a miscarriage, and you cannot foresee the future. Live in this moment and love this stage of your relationship.

Chapter 15
The First Trimester for Baby

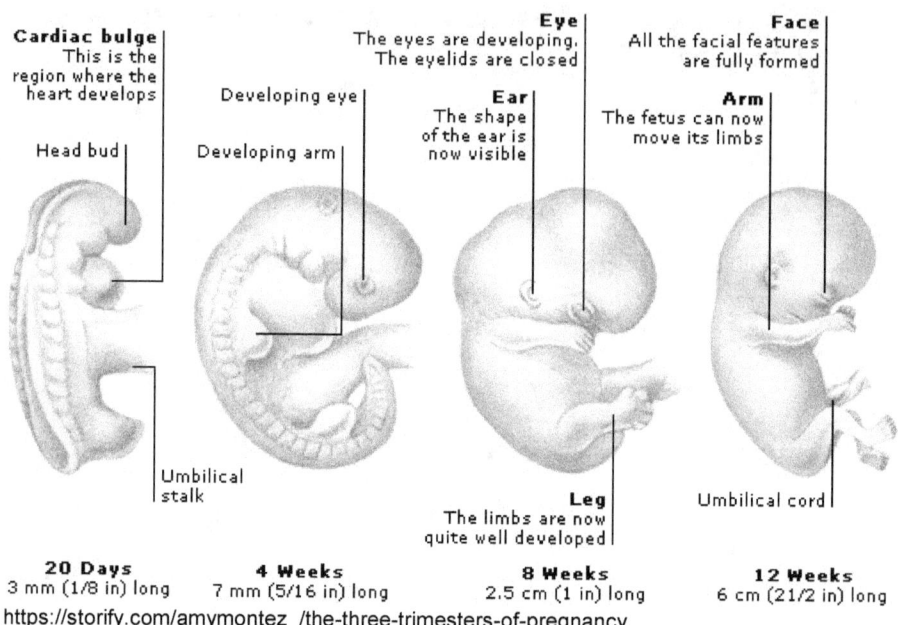

| Cardiac bulge | Eye | Face |
| This is the region where the heart develops | The eyes are developing. The eyelids are closed | All the facial features are fully formed |

Developing eye

Ear
The shape of the ear is now visible

Arm
The fetus can now move its limbs

Head bud

Developing arm

Umbilical stalk

Leg
The limbs are now quite well developed

Umbilical cord

| 20 Days | 4 Weeks | 8 Weeks | 12 Weeks |
| 3 mm (1/8 in) long | 7 mm (5/16 in) long | 2.5 cm (1 in) long | 6 cm (21/2 in) long |

https://storify.com/amymontez /the-three-trimesters-of-pregnancy

It's hard to imagine all that is going on inside your uterus during a pregnancy. Thanks to science, we now know more details than ever before.

HCG is the key hormone present during pregnancy. Its basic job is to tell your body that there is a life growing inside and that your body needs to protect it. Once conception occurs, HCG tells the ovaries to stop producing eggs each month. The level of HCG rises about eight days after ovulation peaks at 60 to 90 days into the pregnancy, and then lowers slightly, leveling off for the remainder of the pregnancy.

Did You Know?

Your baby's sex was determined at conception. The egg and sperm each contribute one chromosome. The egg always carries an X; the sperm, either an X or a Y. If the fertilizing sperm contains an X chromosome, you will have a girl. If it contains a Y, you're having a boy. Although, you will not be able to see the gender until much farther into the pregnancy.

The fertilized egg, also known as a *zygote*, is the size of an apple seed when you can confirm that you're pregnant. Typically, this is about two weeks after conception, so four weeks into the first trimester.

By week five, it has developed into an *embryo*.

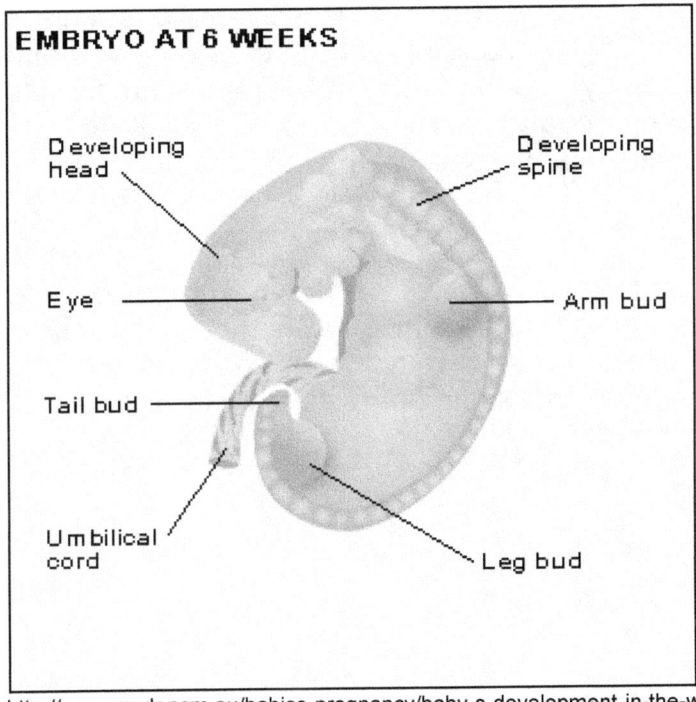

EMBRYO AT 6 WEEKS

Developing head

Developing spine

Eye

Arm bud

Tail bud

Umbilical cord

Leg bud

http://www.mydr.com.au/babies-pregnancy/baby-s-development-in-the-womb

The Embryonic Stage (166)

This stage runs from about the 5th through the 10th week of the first trimester.

As an embryo, all of the baby's major organs and body parts begin to develop. The cells of the embryo, embryonic stem cells, multiply into the hundreds of different types of cells needed to complete a human body.

What is developing now:

Placenta: The placenta is an organ that does not exist unless pregnancy occurs. It is made up of both cells from you and cells from your baby. Its job is the passing of nutrients and sustaining of life through the umbilical cord. I will be talking about the placenta in more detail in the next chapter.

Umbilical cord: The umbilical cord is a ropelike cord connecting the fetus to the placenta. The umbilical cord contains two arteries and a vein, which carry oxygen and nutrients to the fetus and waste products away from the fetus.

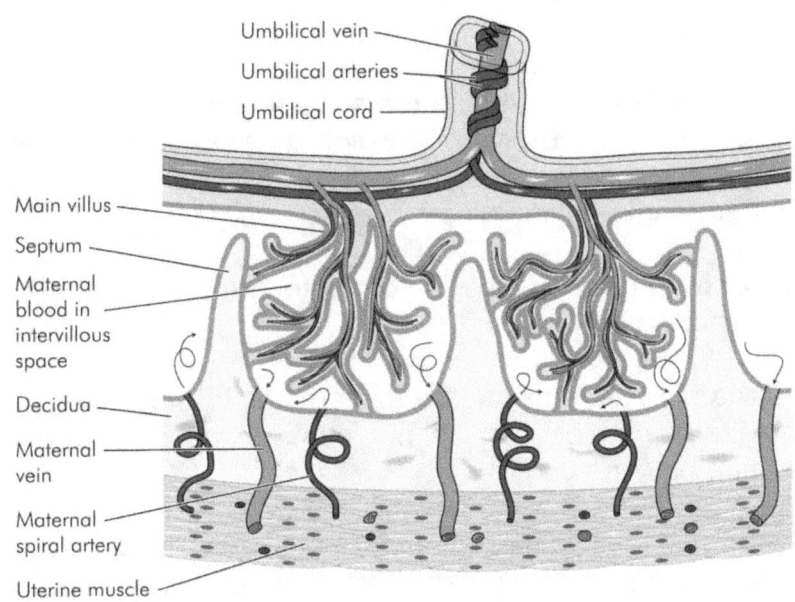

Umbilical vein

Umbilical arteries

Umbilical cord

Main villus

Septum

Maternal blood in intervillous space

Decidua

Maternal vein

Maternal spiral artery

Uterine muscle

Amniotic Sac: This sac is filled with amniotic fluid. It forms inside the uterus to surround and protect the baby. The amniotic fluid is liquid made by both the fetus and the amnion (the membrane that covers the fetal side of the placenta). This sac aids in the musculoskeletal system development and helps to regulate the temperature of the fetus. (167)

Nervous System: One of the first systems to begin development, the nervous system forms the brain, spinal cord, and nerves. (This is why chiropractic is so important to help with balancing the nervous system)

Heart: The baby's heart starts to beat at around 6 weeks. Prior to this, it is an S-shaped tube on the front of the embryo. You may be able to hear or see the baby's heart beat for the first time around 8 weeks pregnant, if you choose to have an early ultrasound exam.

Face: Facial features take shape and the eyes and ears form and are linked to the brain. Eyelids, forehead, nose, nasal passage, cheeks, lips, and jaw all form. The mouth, tooth buds, and tongue all develop.

Arms and Legs: Tiny buds turn into arms and legs with fingers and toes.

Sex Organs: The reproductive system has formed by the end of the first trimester, but it's not possible on ultrasound to determine boy versus girl.

Movement: Muscle development causes twitches and movements, but once the nerves and muscles work together, baby can move with purpose. A mother cannot feel these movements until farther along, as baby is too small at this point.

Growth: By week ten, the embryo is 1-1.5 inches in length.

At eight weeks, the embryo is officially a *fetus* and all organs have been formed.

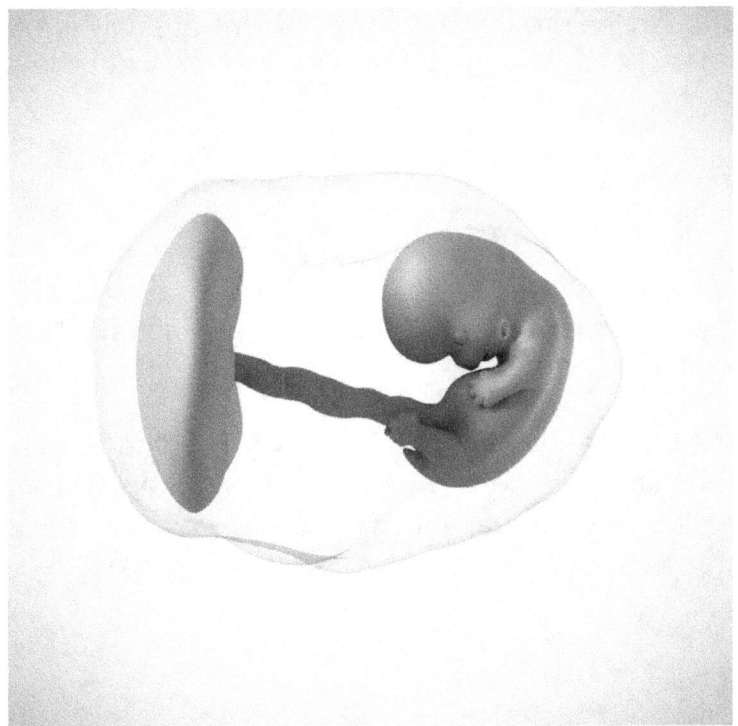

After 10 weeks, the placenta takes charge of producing progesterone and all other hormones. This is known as the Fetal Stage.

The Fetal Stage (166)

Weeks 10, 11 and 12 are the beginning of the fetal stage.
- Fingernails and toenails form.
- Kidneys begin working.
- Movement increases.
- The baby will grow to 3-4 inches in length.

Your baby is the most vulnerable during the first 12 weeks of gestation. Any exposure to drugs, radiation, certain medications, tobacco and toxic substances can potentially cause damage and disrupt normal development.

Even though the organs and body systems are fully formed by the end of 12 weeks, the fetus cannot survive outside of the womb.

Did You Know?

Maternal stress can affect the embryo's development as early as the first trimester.

The first trimester of pregnancy is a crucial time for a baby's hearth health later in life. Research shows that children who are small during the early stages of fetal development are at an increased risk of heart problems once they are older. (168)

Chapter 16
The Amazing Placenta

Most people give little thought to the placenta, and few actually appreciate it.

The placenta is the most unstudied organ. It is a marvelous creation made within the woman's body when pregnancy occurs. Without a placenta, there cannot be future life. For such a small, easily to dispose of organ, a whole lot of life is created. Learning just how important this organ is will help you understand why taking your diet and supplement regimen seriously makes so much sense.

The placenta is unique among organs, critical to life but thrown out as hazardous waste once the baby is born. In its short presence, it serves as a vital protective barrier to the baby. The organ's blood vessels also deliver essential oxygen and nutrients to be passed from the mother. Still, the placenta has been vastly underappreciated. Scientists are taking a closer look and finding that it is much more than hazardous waste: it actively protects the fetus and shapes neurological development. (169)

As soon as three days after fertilization, cells called trophoblasts begin to produce hormones. This is what will become the placenta. These hormones ensure that the lining of the uterus, the endometrium, will be ready for the egg to implant properly. By about five days after fertilization, the trophoblast cells surround the developing embryo and begin to fuse together to form one giant cell with many nuclei. This cell is called the syncytial trophoblast, and its first job is to occupy the uterine and implant firmly.

Over the next few weeks, the developing placenta takes over making the hormones that ensure a healthy pregnancy.

Although implantation has taken part inside of your body, the developing placenta and embryo are not actually part of your body. One of the placenta's most important roles is to protect your baby from an attack by your own immune system. You see, your baby and his placenta are genetically unique and very different from you. (170)

Your blood flows through specific channels within the placenta. When the baby develops his own blood and blood vessels, your blood and the blood of your baby come into close association, but they never mix or come into direct contact. This may surprise you, but a mother and baby generally have different blood types. (171)

The placenta forms a thin, seamless barrier between your blood and your baby's blood. All the important nutrients, hormones, and antibodies that pass from your blood to your baby's must travel across this "sponge." Waste products in your baby's blood must then pass across the placenta to your blood to be disposed of.

While your baby's own organs are maturing, they cannot and do not yet function as they will outside the womb (with exception for the heart). The placenta uses your blood to function as the lungs, kidneys, digestive system, liver, and immune system for the fetus. This is why it is so important to pay attention to what you are consuming while pregnant.

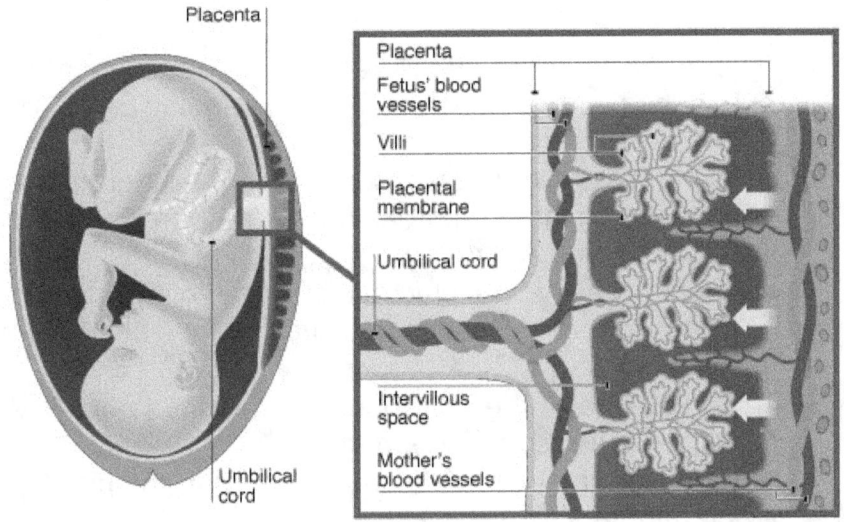

http://www.bbc.co.uk/schools/gcsebitesize/science/add_gateway_pre_2011/living/diffusionr ev2.shtml

The tree-like structures you see in the pictures are called cotyledons. This is how the bloods of both you and your baby stay separated. There are normally 20 of these structures in a mature placenta, and they carry the baby's blood, while the mother's blood flows outside of them. By late pregnancy, the flow of your blood through the placenta reaches a rate of about one pint per minute.

Scientists are still trying to learn how the amazing placenta is not rejected from a mother's body, as it is a "foreign organ" and does not belong to her. What science fails to consider is that a woman's body is designed to carry and birth babies. This is the purpose of our uterus, breasts, and emotionally speaking, our hearts.

Did You Know?

- The placenta grows as the baby grows, reaching about 8-9 inches wide, an inch thick and weighing up to 3lbs at birth.
- The placenta expulsion is known as the afterbirth, or third stage of labor, and can take anywhere from 5-60 minutes to birth after baby.
- Scientists believe the placenta has the ability to predict autism, genetic diseases, premature birth, and preeclampsia. (172)
- The placenta is the only organ that disposes of itself when it's purpose has been met.
- 20% of your blood supply passes through the placenta each minute. *(173)*
- The placenta produces the hormones that signal milk production for the mother, and milk will not be made until the placenta has been fully expelled.
- Identical twins may share a placenta, depending on when the egg splits, or they may have their own.
- Problems with the placenta can lead to preeclampsia, gestational diabetes, prematurity, and stillbirth. (174)
- The placenta can influence lifelong health. Problems can be a marker of later disease for you or your child. (174)

CHAPTER 17
The Second Trimester For Mom

Your body will be physically changing over the next few months, and most moms say that this stage of pregnancy is when they start really bonding with their babies.

Sometime during this trimester, people will actually be able to see that you are pregnant. You may have to ward off strangers wanting to touch your belly; and you may hate your scale.

The adventure of motherhood, or adding a sibling is becoming closer, more tangible. Your hormone levels are balancing, and you actually will have a bit of energy again! Throughout these few months you can expect to experience some (or all) of the following:

Your Body

By the end of the second trimester, the uterus has expanded higher than your belly button. You will breathe faster now because your body has to work harder to keep the level of carbon dioxide in the blood down. Between that and the increased upward pressure on the lungs from your growing baby, no wonder breathing is a little harder!

Lessening of Complaints

- Morning sickness *should* ease up around week 14-15 for most moms. (There are some that experience it throughout the entire pregnancy.)
- Breasts will still be swollen, but they should not be as sore or tender.
- Food aversions may dwindle – and food may taste amazing! Make sure you are getting that protein in!

125

Energy and Happiness

Due to balancing hormones, your mood swings should taper off. You may want to get back into activities that you have ignored the last few months. Take the opportunity to join a prenatal yoga group, jump back on the jogging trails, or dive into the pool.

You are growing big enough to look pregnant, but not big enough to feel uncomfortable. This growth tends to bring a serious bout of happiness with it.

Sex technically equates to more happiness and a more relaxed nature. As you have read, sex is *amazing* during the second trimester! The blood flow and extra sensationalized body tingles enhance the entire experience. Not to mention that your exhaustion has let up, so now you aren't crashing at 6:00pm every night.

Feeling 'Womanly.' You're getting more curves, growing life, glowing from orgasms... it's hard not to feel spectacular. Own it, Mama.

Baby Kicks. You are going to start feeling more and more movements from inside the womb. They will intensify throughout the second trimester. There is nothing better than feeling hiccups and tiny soccer kicks. Your partner will be able to feel them shortly after you can.

New Ailments

While your first trimester woes may be fading, there are a few new things you may experience.

Your breasts may start leaking toward the end of the second trimester. It may happen in the third trimester – or not at all. None of these timeframes reflect your milk supply – or play a role in your breastfeeding journey! Do not worry if you never leak milk.

Food cravings may kick in for things you have never even tasted before. New flavors or more intense ones may be just what this baby is enjoying!

Heartburn tends to flare up from now until the end of pregnancy, but that may have something to do with your food cravings – or not, it may just be part of your pregnancy. Review my heartburn remedies for relief.

Leg Cramps may be sneaking up on you. Ease them by adding more magnesium into your life through baths, lotions, or supplements. Staying hydrated, active, and seeing your chiropractor should help too.

UTI's are more common during the second trimester. Make sure you let your birth team know if you are experiencing them.

Swelling shouldn't be painful or so noticeable yet, but it may happen on days you are standing a lot. Rest, eat healthy, and stay hydrated. If you notice sudden swelling, head in to your doctor for a blood pressure test to rule preeclampsia out.

Constipation is common at this point in pregnancy. Up your fiber and water intake each day for some relief.

Skin Changes such as Melasma, the pregnancy mask, may appear along with the development of the linea nigra, which is the dark line from the belly button all the way down (or up) the stomach. *Stretch marks* may also start popping up.

Weight Gain. You will (and should) be slowly gaining weight right now. There is no perfect number you should see on the scale, in fact, ditch the scale altogether. Let your doctor weigh you at appointments and just maintain a healthy lifestyle and enjoy this pregnancy!

Ligament pains can be quite intense for some women. See your prenatal chiropractor regularly.

Braxton Hicks Contractions are common and good for the baby and uterus. These are like training exercises for the big day of labor. They feel like a tight band around your expanding belly.

Daydreaming

This is typically the time that you want to start shopping and sharing your pregnancy out loud. Let your mind race and run wild. Make lists of baby names, write letters to your baby, and plan new traditions.

Planning

- Start talking, reading, and educating yourself about birth.

- Register for a real birth class beyond what is offered at the hospital. Some series are 12 weeks long and should be started toward the end of the second trimester – and many may have a waiting list, so call now.

- Talk to your employer if you have not done so yet, and set up your maternity leave plan.

- Sign up for your hospital or birth center tour, and prepare a list of questions so that you will leave knowing every little thing that will (or could) occur during your stay.

- Register for anything you'd like to receive or purchase for the baby and start working on a nursery, if you would like one.

This is also the time to talk to friends about a baby shower, and pick a date.

Appointments

Your doctor or midwife visits are still every 4 weeks, but you will be able to find and hear the baby's heartbeat with ease during them now. As baby grows, your doctor will help you figure out his current position and decipher between a foot and an arm kicking you.

The big appointment most moms refer during this trimester is known as the 20 week ultrasound. This is when (if you choose) you learn the baby's gender, find out if everything is developing as it should, and that both you and baby are healthy. It is also an appointment that you may learn of any potential troubles, so it can be an emotional experience for couples.

Toward the end of the second trimester, your doctor or midwife will ask you to start thinking about your birth. It can be an overwhelming and frightening thing to plan for, so starting now to work through your emotions is a good idea.

Did You Know?

Most partners love this stage of pregnancy. You have more energy, and they can begin to physically see the changes that pregnancy brings. Most partners feel a stronger attraction to you during this point in pregnancy too!

CHAPTER 18
The Second Trimester for Baby

Gestational weeks 13-27 make up the second trimester.

What is happening inside your womb right now?

What started as a cluster of cells has continued multiplying and grown into a fetus. There are functioning organs, nerves, and muscles now. The heartbeat can now be heard easily with a Doppler at your appointments.
Remember that every pregnancy and baby is different, so your baby may develop a bit quicker or slower than this timeline. Trust in your ability to grow and nurture this baby while he is inside of you.

Week 13

- The placenta and umbilical cord are now providing oxygen and nutrients for your baby. Baby is using breathing movements by utilizing the amniotic fluid to practice 'breathing' in and out.
- Their heart is still beating fast; faster than it will towards the end of pregnancy and after she is born.
- Tissue that will become bone is developing in the head and throughout the arms and legs.
- Baby's ears and eyes are still developing and will continue to move forward on the head into their permanent places.
- The skin is covered in a fine hair called lanugo.
- Neck is lengthening.
- Hands and fingers are becoming functional, meaning they can suck their thumb.

Week 14

- Not only is your baby 'practice-breathing' amniotic fluid, but they are now 'drinking' it as well. This is how the muscles learn to work once introduced to the real world, they practice with the amniotic fluid.
- They can urinate. Yes, your baby can now pee. The intestines have moved from the umbilical cord to the abdomen. Urine can form and be dispensed back into the amniotic fluid.
- Baby may be able to hear you. The middle ear bones are hardening.
- Red blood cells are forming in the spleen.
- Your baby's sex will become apparent this week (or in the coming weeks). Ovarian follicles form or the prostate appears.
- Now about 3.5 inches long.

Week 15

- Your baby's scalp and hair pattern are forming.
- The legs are longer than their arms, and they are now large enough for you to *possibly* start feeling him use them to kick!
- The skin is still very thin and opaque, but the fingernails and toenails are growing.

Week 16

- An ultrasound would show you just how intense your baby's movements are right now! Baby is flipping and marching all over in there – maybe you can feel them moving.

- Eyes are now facing forward.
- Fat is beginning to form under the skin, and the neck is strengthening.
- She is sucking, swallowing, and blinking throughout the days now.
- Baby is measuring around 4.5 inches.

Week 17

- The umbilical cord thickens and there is possible meconium backing up in the bowels.
- Tissue continues hardening to bone.
- You may feel little hiccups!
- Fat continues accumulating, which will help to regulate baby's body temperature after birth.
- Baby is now just over 5 inches long.

Week 18

- Vernix begins to form over the skin.
- The placenta continues to grow.
- The lungs and vocal cords develop alveoli.
- The gender is more accurately predicted by ultrasound at this point or afterward.
- Your baby may start to react to sounds or voices outside the womb.
- Now over 5.5 inches in length.

Week 19

- A baby girl's uterus and vagina are forming.

- Their permanent teeth are forming behind the baby teeth that are already under the gums.
- They begin sleeping on the same (or similar) schedule they will follow as a newborn.
- Now measures just over 6 inches in length.

Week 20

- The half-way point!
- 80-90% of babies reveal their gender through ultrasound this week.
- The uterus is continually expanding to accommodate your baby.
- Growth begins to slow down around this week and level out to an even growth rate for the remainder of pregnancy.
- Nerve cells are developing to experience new senses.
- Measureing about 6.5 inches in length from crown to rump, but measurements at this point are taken from the crown of the head to heel of the foot, so she'll average about 10 inches in length.

Week 21

- Your baby's white blood cells begin to form.
- Skin is still opaque, and they are now swallowing easily.
- Tongue is developing.

Week 22

- The fine hair (Lanugo) is now fully covering your baby. (This helps keeps the vernix on)
- Eyelids and eyebrows are complete.
- A boy baby is forming sperm and testosterone, with his testes moving into place.
- Your baby may be close to weighing a pound now.

Week 23

- Your baby's body proportions are almost normal now.
- Eyes are fully formed, but they do not have color yet.
- Skin is wrinkled and fingerprints are forming.
- A girl's ovaries now hold a lifetime supply of eggs.

Week 24

- Your baby's real hair is growing, unless she is meant to be a bald baby. Both outcomes are normal.
- The taste buds of the tongue are continuing to develop, as are the lungs.
- The baby is now officially viable, meaning she has a chance at surviving outside the womb *with medical help* now. She will have a 15% chance of survival. This percentage increases each day she is in the womb.
- Rapid Eye Movement (REM) occurs during her sleep cycles.
- Measuring about 11 inches long.

Week 25

- Your baby's position and movements put intense pressure on your bladder, causing frequent bathroom trips and making for unpleasant sleep positions.
- Your baby's spine is still forming and his nostrils are now opening.
- They can wiggle his fingers and toes.
- Baby is just over 13.5 inches long and close to a pound and a half in weight.

Week 26

- Your baby's lungs are beginning to produce surfactant, the substance that allows the air sacs in the lungs to inflate.
- Finger and toenails are complete.
- Retinas are formed and they can open their eyes and blink.
- There are detectable brain waves in response to hearing and sight.
- Measuring about 14 inches long.

Week 27

- During the last week of the second trimester, your baby's lungs and nervous system are continuing to mature.
- Your baby is about 14.5 inches long.

(175)(176)(177)

CHAPTER 19
Alternatives to Standard Gestational Diabetes Testing

You will soon be presented with taking the gestational diabetes test. You hear many women laugh the test and the condition off as if it is just another common ailment in pregnancy. Our society tends to do this too often. The chemical-filled, sweet drink so many women think is mandatory – IS NOT. First, nothing is mandatory. Second, that drink should not consumed by anyone!

There are options. Declining the test all together is an option, but not an option that most would take. But that does not mean you need to partake in the drink style of testing.

According to the American Pregnancy Association:
"Pregnant women can develop a condition known as Gestational Diabetes (diabetes brought on by pregnancy) which can pose a risk to both mother and baby. A glucose tolerance test is a common type of testing for potential gestational diabetes."

Gestational Diabetes

Typically, the body breaks down carbohydrates into glucose causing insulin to be released. The insulin pulls the glucose from the blood and transfers it to the cells to be stored for energy. When a woman is pregnant, the body leaves some glucose in the blood so that it can be passed to the baby through the placenta and umbilical cord.

Gestational Diabetes is diagnosed when there is too high of an amount of glucose found in the blood while pregnant.

Science has not found one specific cause for gestational diabetes, but the following are all possible links:

- Overeating
- Excess Carbohydrate or Sugar Consumption
- Stress
- Autoimmune Issues
- Sleep Deprivation

The Dangers and Complications of Gestational Diabetes: (178)
- Increased C-section Rates
- Increased NICU visits
- Birth Injuries (Such as shoulder dystocia)
- Large Babies: Although over 70% of 'Large Babies' are born to mothers without gestational diabetes, women with the condition have been linked to having above average-sized babies.
- Neonatal Hypoglycemia: low blood sugar in baby. (179)
- Fetal Hyperinsulinemia: the baby has higher levels of insulin after birth due to receiving too much glucose while in the womb.
- Jaundice
- Preeclampsia
- Increased risk of the mother developing type 2 diabetes later in life

How is Gestational Diabetes Diagnosed?

Signs of Gestational Diabetes Include: (178)
- Sugar in urine
- Unusual thirst
- Frequent urination
- Fatigue
- Nausea
- Frequent vaginal, bladder, and skin infections
- Blurred vision

It has become common practice for every pregnant woman to be tested for gestational diabetes, even though it is unclear just how accurate results are. One study shows that insulin naturally increases throughout pregnancy, and throughout the day. (180)

This means that the results you are given are dependent on the gestational week of your pregnancy and the time of day you were tested. It is unclear if this test is truly necessary, as only about 5% of pregnant women will be diagnosed. (332)

Current guidelines recommend what is called a "two step approach" for screening for gestational diabetes. The first step is a glucose challenge test (GCT).   During the GCT, the woman is given Glucola, a sugar drink, and then has her blood sugar level tested one hour after consuming said drink. If the results are above the normal range, the woman will come back to perform a 3-hour version of the test. (182)

Glucola: The Drink

Glucola includes ingredients such as brominated oil (BVO), food   dyes,   sodium   benzonate,   BHA,   sodium hexametaphosphate,   dextrose,   and   'natural flavorings.' Preservatives and food dyes alone are enough to avoid the drink while pregnant, but the
BVO (banned in Japan and Europe) can accumulate in the organs of the body and potentially cause heart lesions, changes in the liver, and alter behavioral development.(333) It has even been found in the breastmilk of mothers who drink sodas or sugar drinks that contain BVO (Many companies are withdrawing the ingredient from their products). This 'oil' has been linked to neurological problems, fertility problems, changes in thyroid hormones and early puberty.

This drink should not be recommended for consumption for anyone, especially to a pregnant woman. (154)

Alternative Test Options

Instead of consuming Glucola, these options may be more appealing:

- 50 GM of Organic Grape Juice (or apple juice)
- 50 GM of Jelly Beans (About 50 beans): Of course, reach for the non-GMO, naturally colored version
- 50g of Glucolift: This is a natural, non-GMO, artificial colors & flavors free glucose tablet. It's made for people with type 1 diabetes who need to raise their blood sugar regularly throughout the day. (Many midwives will have this available)
- 50 GM Breakfast Meal: This can consist of several options so talk to your birth team or research which you would most prefer before presenting the idea to your doctor.

Meals typically include eggs, juice, toast, and fruit, but some midwives or doctors include pancakes! It is harder to be exact with glucose levels of real food, but the body processes real food the easiest and will give you the least chances of any stomach aches afterward.

Make sure you talk with your birth team, as they may have other alternatives available as well!

Asking to Skip the Drink

Your birth team should fully support your decisions throughout your pregnancy. No doctor has the right to tell you that you _must_ perform or complete something. If you experience resistance from your doctor about selecting an alternative glucose testing option, your best stance to take is an educated one.

The placenta is not a filter, but a sponge. You know how harmful chemicals can be, so why is it ok to agree to drink them? These chemicals will be passed to the baby. Common sense says this is not right. Once you factor in the side effects and chances of an inaccurate test result, your doctor should support your alternative decision.

<u>The ACOG clearly states that doctors must respect their patients' decisions and that each pregnant woman is an individual and has the right for unique standard of care.</u>

CHAPTER 20
Managing Gestational Diabetes

The American Diabetes Association states that there is no known cure for gestational diabetes, but that treating the condition is done in two ways: *Diet and Exercise.*

Even if you are required to monitor your glucose levels daily and/or administer insulin shots, you will still be asked to follow a specific diet and increase your exercise level. (Talk to your midwife or doctor, and do plenty of research, before you decide to administer insulin shots daily during pregnancy.)

The world can be a very overwhelming and confusing place when it comes to diet and exercise, but now you are trying to figure it all out while juggling a pregnancy and gestational diabetes.

First, if there is glucose in your urine, you are not guaranteed to have gestational diabetes. You may just need monitoring and to follow-up with future testing. Whether you have been diagnosed with gestational diabetes or you are trying to prevent it, diet and exercise are your best friends. As a chiropractor, I encourage all moms to follow a healthy lifestyle before, during, and after pregnancy, but the following ideas may give you a better understanding of how to do just that.

I'm going to break down the diet and exercise into easy to manage ideas that you can incorporate into your daily life without feeling deprived, and at the same time lower your chances of having a c-section. Remember to consult your personal midwife or doctor before altering your lifestyle drastically.

Exercise

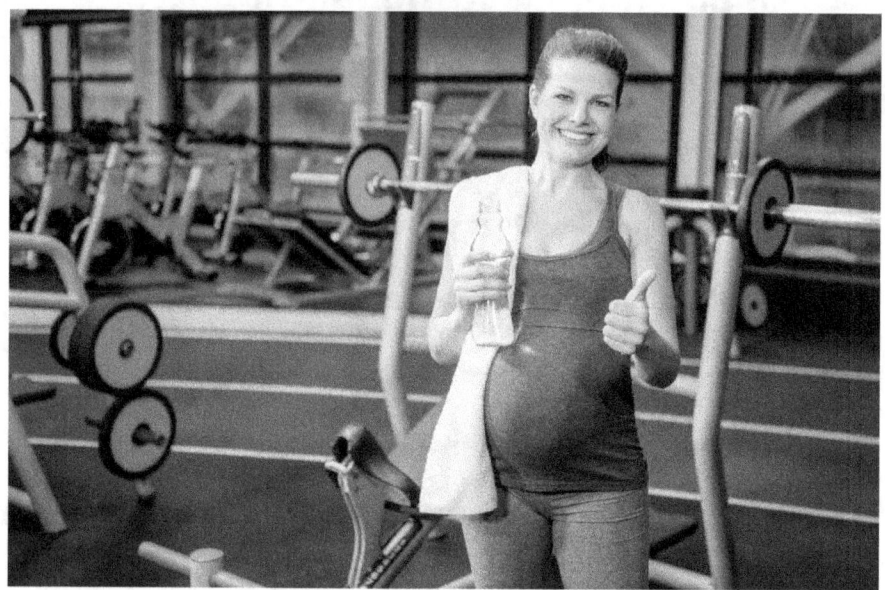

GET MOVING!

One hour of exercise each day, even broken into two 30 minute sessions is sufficient to help raise the heartrate enough for the body to manage weight gain, prevent or manage gestational diabetes, and help maintain a healthy pregnancy overall.(183)

While walking technically is exercise, you need to make sure that it is more than a leisurely stroll. The body doesn't truly recognize your normal walking pace as needing an increased heartrate.

Great ways to exercise pregnant:
- Continue your normal exercise routine, if you have been active.
- Enroll in prenatal classes, such as bootcamps, yoga, aerobics, or basic prenatal fitness.

- Walk farther and quicker than your leisurely pace, trying to break a small sweat.
- Swimming
- Biking
- Hiking
- Elliptical or other stationary equipment
- Strength Training with or without weights

Diet

The Standard American Diet (SAD) is not exactly up to par. It's easy to see just why so many people are experiencing conditions such as gestational diabetes. We are addicted to sugar and other foods that break down into sugar. We cannot let go of dairy or pesticide-sprayed gluten and wheat. We can't put down the GMO-filled, processed products. But we are suffering. Not only are we suffering, but our children are too – even in utero.

A few rules to follow:

- *DROP ALL PROCESSED FOODS.* If it comes in a box or bag, drop it.

- *Stay away from sugar.* Look for hidden sugar. Yogurt is known for a ton of "hidden Sugar!" Here is how to calculate for hidden sugar:

This is for a small strawberry yogurt you would find store and given to children in school.

Add Sugar + Carbohydrates – Fiber = Total Sugar Grams

Example: 19+20-0(no fiber)= 39g total sugar

That's a lot of sugar, and this is yogurt is advertised as a health choice. Again, the SAD needs improvement.

- *Eat every 2-3 hours – including a midnight snack.* It is recommended to eat small meals every 2-3 hours so your body becomes used to processing and absorbing nutrients regularly, which helps to prevent the highs and lows of blood sugar levels that characterize diabetes.

- *Keep carbohydrates to a minimum* and eat them in the middle of the day so that you are not consuming hem before sleep. Complex carbohydrates are more valuable. Eliminating simple carbohydrates could help prevent or treat gestational diabetes.

- *Increase your protein with The Brewer's Diet.* One of the important functions of protein is to help break down carbohydrates. Eating at least 75-120g of protein a day is essential. If you are eating whole-food carbohydrates, pair them with proteins. This will help to utilize only the necessary amounts of insulin.

- *Increase your fiber.* Fiber can provoke the activity of insulin receptors and can also prevent the release of excess insulin into the bloodstream. This helps to balance the levels of insulin and avoid the onset of diabetes. (183)

- *Eat healthy snacks*: Green leafy vegetables and fruit have been shown to prevent gestational diabetes. (184)

Foods to include:
- Flaxseed

- Brewer's Yeast (natural chromium)
- Eggs: high in choline, which helps promote baby's growth and brain development.
- Whole Fat Yogurt: avoid added fruits and sugars
- Grass Fed Meat
- Grass Fed Butter
- Avocados
- Wild Caught Fish
- Tomatoes: The main antioxidant in tomatoes is Lycopene, which has been linked to the reduction of preeclampsia.
- Sweet Potatoes: Full of antioxidants, vitamins A, C and B6, folate and fiber
- Dark, Leafy Greens: Full of antioxidants, vitamins and minerals. Spinach is also a great source of non-dairy calcium and fiber.
- Beans: Full of fiber, protein, folate, iron, calcium and zinc.
- Nuts
- Berries
- Citrus Fruits
- Pears
- Broccoli
- Cabbage
- Mushrooms
- Peppers
- Onions
- Green Beans
- Olives
- Lentils
- Oats
- Quinoa
- Okra
- Carrots
- Chia Seeds
- Fats/Oils: animal fats, coconut oil, olive oil, olives, avocados, fish oils, etc. should be high quality.

Note that some fruit and vegetables effect blood sugar levels more than others. For example, the following are 'heavier' and denser foods and should be eaten with protein.

- Ripe Bananas
- Melon
- Pineapple
- Apples

Foods to Avoid:

- White Foods - White potatoes, white rice, white bread, white pasta.
- Candy, Cookies, Cakes – Sweets in general.
- Processed Products: Processed, packaged, and most restaurant food quality is impossible to predict.

Supplements to Consider

(Again, talk to your doctor before adding or altering your diet or supplements.)

- Vitamin D (185)
- Vitamin C: Ascorbic acid has the ability to influence glucose tolerance.(186)

- Chromium – This is used up whenever sugar or flour is digested. It naturally runs low in the third trimester, but an unhealthy diet completely depletes it faster. (Some people have seen drastic results in their glucose numbers with two weeks of supplementing with chromium.) (334)

- Inositol- studies show improved insulin sensitivity and decreased glucose levels with the use of inositol while pregnant. (187)

- Astragalus - Research shows that astragalus (along with traditional treatments for gestational diabetes) is linked to significantly better blood sugar control and milder symptoms of gestational diabetes. (188)

- Berberine - It has been shown to regulate glucose and lipid metabolism in vitro. It significantly lowers cholesterol, FBG and PBG.(335) http://www.ncbi.nlm.nih.gov/pmc/articles/PMC2410097/

Chapter 21
Sonograms and Ultrasounds

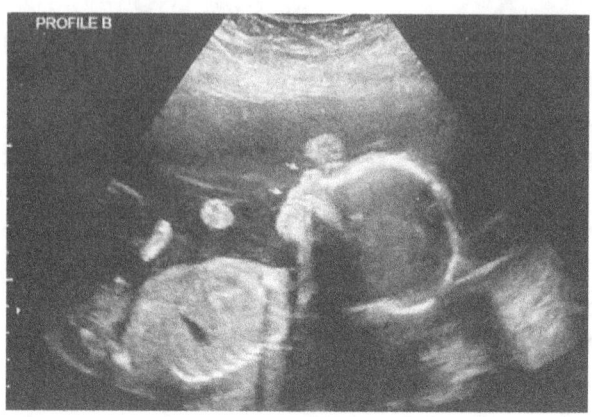

There is something so exciting about seeing your baby bouncing around on the ultrasound screen, but is it safe for you or your baby?

The truth is that scientists have uncovered evidence suggesting that ultrasound scans on pregnant women can increase the risk of decreased fetal growth, leading to low birth weight (189) and possibly cause subtle brain damage in their unborn babies, especially with boys. In 2006, a study was done utilizing pregnant mice and ultrasonography. The results: Frequent use of ultrasound caused brain abnormalities in the developing fetuses of these mice. (190)

Research published in 2016 has identified that the exposure to first trimester ultrasounds is linked to decreased non-verbal IQ and increased repetitive behaviors 'relative to male children with ASD.' (336)
While research is being continued, there is enough to know not to allow excessive scans throughout your pregnancy. Remember that you have the ultimate say in your prenatal care!

Healthy, low-risk pregnant women are recommended to receive only one sonogram, near 20 weeks gestation. Even this scan is recommended to be done in a timely manner. But, on average, women receive 4.55 ultrasounds per pregnancy. This is far too many, as research shows that scans performed 5 times throughout the pregnancy are linked to low birth weight. (337)

However, 20% of pregnancies are 'high risk' and there may be times when cause arises and other scans are recommended by your birth team to check on your baby. Always perform your own research to learn your options.

In this chapter, I'm going to break down each type of sonogram and explain their individual purposes and what you will learn if you decide to have one.

Before describing the sonograms, let's talk about the difference between a sonogram and an ultrasound.

A sonogram is the image produced during an ultrasound (the picture you see and get to take home), and the ultrasound is technique that uses sound waves above what we can hear (about 20 kHz) to see or hear inside the body. (191)

There are several ultrasounds that may be mentioned to you:

- Standard Ultrasound
- Advanced Ultrasound
- Doppler Ultrasound
- 3-D Ultrasound
- 4-D or Dynamic 3-D Ultrasound
- Fetal Echocardiography (Used when congenital heart defects are suspected.)

Your doctor or midwife will likely use the Doppler during each prenatal visit past 10/12 weeks to pick up your baby's heartbeat. It's done quick and easy, without being invasive at all. It is still an ultrasound though, meaning sound waves are present. You can of course deny this and ask for a stethoscope to be used instead. (A stethoscope is easier to use the farther you are in the pregnancy.)

Your doctor or midwife may recommend one or more of the following sonograms throughout your pregnancy, for various reasons.

Dating Scan: (192) A dating scan is an ultrasound done trans-vaginally (the ultrasound wand will be inserted into your vagina) to establish the gestational age of the pregnancy. You will see the start of a pregnancy as early as 4 weeks and 3 days along (but some pregnancy cannot be seen until 5 weeks). This scan can show the beginnings of a gestational sac, but no heartbeat or further fetal development yet at this stage. An embryo and heartbeat can be seen (not heard) as early as 6 weeks and 3 days, but may not be picked up until further along. You will also learn the location of your pregnancy. If there is a chance that it is ectopic, you will find out now.

- A dating scan can determine the number of gestational sacs present (if there is more than one, it may be reabsorbed by the end of the 1st trimester). Your cervix, uterus position, and ovaries will also be seen, and you will learn if there is any visible clotting or possible neural tube defects. (193)
- A sonogram produced at 9 weeks or earlier will be the most accurate to use for dating the pregnancy.

- Breakdown of what can be seen according to Advanced Women's Imaging: (194)
    - at 5 ½ weeks gestation a tiny sac can be seen in the uterus, but the baby and its heart beat may not be detected yet.

    - By 6 to 7 weeks gestation the embryo and heart beat can be seen (Heartbeat will be about 90 to 110 beats per minute under 6 to 7 weeks, then 110 to 200 beats per minute as the baby matures, possibly slowing down a bit toward the end of pregnancy).

- o By 8 weeks gestation the baby and its heart beat can be found through an abdominal ultrasound.

1st Trimester Scan (Also known as a NT Scan): Having a transabdominal ultrasound between 10-14 weeks is done to confirm your baby's heart beat and perform elected first trimester screening (called a 'combined test') for chromosomal abnormalities. The screening is optional for one or all of the following: Down's syndrome (Trisomy 21 or T21), Edwards' syndrome (Trisomy 18 or T18) and Patau's syndrome (Trisomy 13 or T13). The combined test involves a blood test and an ultrasound scan. If a screening test shows that you have a higher risk of having a baby with Down's, Edwards' or Patau's syndromes, you will be offered diagnostic tests to find out for certain if your baby has the condition.

- The nuchal translucency (NT Scan) portion of the test can identify other significant abnormalities, such as cardiac disorders. The screening test does not detect neural tube defects. With an accuracy rate of 85%, and a false positive rate of 5%, a positive test means you have a 1/100 to 1/300 chance of experiencing one of the abnormalities. (195) (196)

Anomaly Scan (20 week Ultrasound): This is the one recommended ultrasound that each pregnant woman received. It can be done between 18-21 weeks, and includes a more in-depth ultrasound to determine the baby's size, weight and growth measurements.

Any signs of abnormal growth should be found during this scan. The following fetal parts are measured and checked during the anatomy ultrasound: (197)

- o Face: Depending on the positioning of your baby, the technician may or may not be able to detect if your baby has a cleft lip.
- o Brain: The technician will be measuring the fluid-filled spaces inside the brain and the shape of the cerebellum, which is in the back of the brain. Any cysts should be seen, which may indicate a slightly increased risk for a chromosome abnormality.
- o Skull
- o Neck
- o Spine: The technician will be looking to make sure that the vertebrae are in alignment and that the skin covers the spine at the back.
- o Heart (rate, rhythm, 4-chambers, and outflow): Congenital Heart Defects are one of the leading causes of birth defects and infant death.
- o Lungs
- o Abdomen (stomach, kidneys, liver, bladder, umbilicus cord)
- o Limbs
- o Genitals

Your placenta positioning will be looked at as well as your cervix position. (198)

Level II Scan: While technically the above mentioned anatomy scan is a Level II scan, there are other reasons to need a Level II sonogram. Level II scans are reserved for high-risk mothers.

Biophysical Attribute	Normal	Abnormal
Breathing	1 breathing episode within 30 minutes	No breathing episodes within 30 minutes
Movement	2 or more movements within 30 minutes	less than 2 movements within 30 minutes
Muscle Tone	1 or more episodes of active extension/flexion of limbs, etc. (i.e. opening and closing a hand).	Slow extension/flexion of limbs, partially open fetal hand, etc
Heart Rate	2 or more episodes of reactive heart rate acceleration within 20 min	1 or more episodes of unreactive heart rate acceleration
Amniotic Fluid	1 or more adequate pockets of fluid	Either no pockets or inadequate pockets of fluid

Family history of birth defects, maternal medical problems, exposure to certain medications, a maternal age of 35 or older, abnormal screening results, and suspected birth defects are all reason for this scan.

A survey of your baby's internal organs will be conducted, as well as

- o The umbilical cord
- o Amniotic fluid
- o Location of the placenta
- o Fetal heart rate

BPP Scan (Biophsyical Profile): This sonogram combines an ultrasound with a non-stress test (NST) and determines fetal health during the third trimester. The NST involves attaching two belts to your abdomen, one to measure fetal heart rate, and another to measure contractions. Movement and heart rate are measured for 20-30 minutes. Five specific fetal attributes are studied and "scored" during the BPP. (American Pregnancy Association. Biophysical Profile (199).)

NST Scan: The Fetal Non-Stress Test is a non-invasive test performed in pregnancies_over 28 weeks gestation. As mentioned above, The NST involves attaching a belt to the mother's abdomen to measure fetal heart rate, and another belt to measure contractions. A NST may be performed if:
- o Your baby is not moving as much as normal
- o You are overdue
- o There is any reason to suspect the placenta is not functioning adequately
- o You are high risk

The test will show fetal distress, such as the baby not receiving enough oxygen.

The main purpose of the test is to measure the heart rate of your baby in response to his own movements. Healthy babies will have an increased heart rate during times of movement, and the heart rate will decrease afterward.(200)

Chapter 22

3rd Trimester for the Mom

Before you know it, you will be rounding the corner and heading into the final trimester of your pregnancy. Beginning the 28th week, you will see your birth team every two weeks for appointments, until week 36, when you should be seen weekly. Your midwife will be taking fundal height measurements, listening to the heartbeat, and by 32 weeks, she should be able to feel your baby's position. You may also enjoy belly mapping yourself to determine where baby is in there! www.spinningbabies.com is a great resource for belly mapping and positions for baby. Do not panic if your baby is not head down and engaged yet, there is plenty of time.

If your doctor gives the option of checking your cervix for progress before labor begins, please don't let your curiosity get the better of you. Cervical checks are not an indication of impending labor, but they can potentially disrupt your pregnancy.

Throughout weeks 28-42, you may experience much of the following:

New Emotions

You may begin 'nesting' and feel a need to accomplish quite a few things before your baby makes his appearance. This is common, but it can feel overwhelming. Make yourself a master list of what you would like done and work away at it over days or weeks.

There are a lot of feelings you will work through during the third trimester, feelings over:

- Upcoming labor and birth

- Motherhood (or adding a sibling)
- Maternity Leave
- Caring for a Newborn

If you are feeling overly anxious, sad or depressed, please reach out to your birth team; they will have resources to help you work through your feelings.

Many women feel less attractive and more self-conscious during this time period. Ask your partner for support in this area, as you are a *beautiful* woman growing this baby!

Talk to friends and your partner often about your feelings. Write about them even. Taking a supportive birthing and newborn class will also help you feel more prepared and less anxious.

Body Changes

You are feeling more and more 'pregnant' with each passing week. Your belly is also growing more and more each week. Eating high quality, healthy foods is still very important, as is getting as much rest as possible. Exercise can be continued throughout the duration of the pregnancy as long as you are feeling good. Listen to your body, it will tell you what is right for you.

Along with extra weight, you may experience your first trimester symptoms again. I know that sounds miserable, and it may be, but there is a light at the end of the tunnel now. It won't be long until your baby comes earthside.

The most common third trimester ailments include: (201) (202)

Backaches: You are carrying more weight and will start to feel it. Talk to your chiropractor about how you are feeling.

Braxton Hicks Contractions: These will become more frequent as you progress through the third trimester. If you are experiencing them regularly at more than 6 an hour, call your doctor. Laying down, taking a relaxing bath, or just resting for a while should end them.

Dry or Itchy Skin: Stay hydrated and moisturize the skin as often as needed.

Exhaustion: The body is working hard to finish growing this baby. Ask for help if needed so that you can close your eyes at some point during the day.

Feeling Hot: Increased body temperature will cause you to wear less clothing.

Frequent Urination: Again, the organs are all being compressed right now. This, combined with a growing baby who likes to 'tap dance on the bladder' may send you running to the bathroom more often.

Groin Pain: Heavy pressure, pulls, pinches, tweaks, dull aches, and sharp quick pains are all par for the course right now. Your baby is positioning herself for birth and your body is accommodating. Extreme pain should be brought to your birth team's attention.

Heartburn: Eat small, frequent meals and drink plenty of water. Elevate your upper body while resting or sleeping and avoid bending over or lying down after a meal.

Hemorrhoids: Avoid straining to have a bowel movement, and remember to do your kegels! Aloe Vera gel is great for cooling and inflammation.

Increased Discharge: Vaginal discharge may increase.

Leaking Breasts: Colostrum may begin leaking. (Remember that this is not needed for a successful breastfeeding relationship.)

Leg Cramps: Increase your magnesium, calcium and water intake! This is most common in the evening or middle of the night.

Mucus Plug: Losing the mucus plug does not mean that labor will start. It can regrow. However, if you are nearing your estimated due date, it could be a sign that things may progress over the next few days. (Again, it can also mean nothing!)

Shortness of Breath: The uterus is rapidly expanding and compressing against the other organs of the body. Practice good posture, visit your chiropractor, and work on deeper breathing.

Stretch Marks: They may wait until the day before labor to appear (if they appear at all), or you may already see them. The good news is that after birth, the stretch marks will fade from purple or red to a tan or white.

Trouble Sleeping: It is hard to get comfortable as your belly grows larger. A body pillow is helpful, but your best bet is to make sure you are really tired. Exercising should help; it will ensure that you have exerted all of your energy. Your chiropractor may provide you with some relief as well.

One thing to note is that handling any insomnia you may encounter during this time reduces the risk of postpartum depression once baby is born. Remember that exercise, a healthy diet, letting go of stress, and working with your chiropractor can all help in successfully beating insomnia. (203)

The 'Lightening'

At the very end of pregnancy, you may experience something called the lightening. Some refer to it as the baby dropping, and many believe that it is a sign that labor is near. While you may not feel anything, you may find that you can suddenly consume more food and breathe a little easier.

Preparing for Birth

You should be already attending or beginning your birth classes now. Remember that the earlier you begin preparing for labor, the more time you have to work on your relaxation techniques and emotional readiness to give birth.

Pack your birth bag, or prepare your homebirth kit, by week 35 or 36. While most women reach their approximate due date (or surpass it), some go into labor earlier.

Use the time you have left before baby arrives to mentally prepare for labor and newborn care.

Birth Bag List

Many of these items are specific to certain places of birth. Remember that every mother (and birth) is different, so a lot of the items may or may not appeal to you. Pass no judgement, as another mother may want them.

For The Midwife: (Homebirth)

A supply list will be provided from your midwife

- Sterile Gloves
- Waterproof Flashlight
- Large Bowl
- Baking Sheet (to lay tools on)
- Heating Pad and Pillow Case (The pillow case holds the heat source and is used to keep baby warm)
- Emergency Contact Phone Number List
- Tarps, plastic shower curtains, waterproof layers to lay down (Waterproof mattress cover should already be in place)
- Large Towels
- Snacks/Food

For The Mom:

- Your Birth Plan
- Arnica (Other homeopathics too)
- Chux Pads (Various Sizes)
- Hibiclens
- Tucks Pads with Witch Hazel
- Peri Bottle
- New Mom Spray (Earth Mama brand is my favorite!)
- Olive or Coconut Oil
- Water Thermometer (Ensure birth tub is not too hot)
- Heavy Flow Overnight Pads
- Underwear (Full- cut)
- Birth Ball
- Mirror (for birth, not makeup)
- Hair Ties
- Chap Stick
- Water Bottle
- Food/Snacks
- Flip Flops
- Music

- Essential Oils
- Nursing Nightgown
- Robe
- Favorite Pillow
- Sitz Bath
- Nursing Bra (Soft, no under-wire)
- Shower Supplies (Toothbrush and all)
- Breastfeeding Pillow
- Loose fitting, soft clothes
- Rebozo
- Rice Sock
- Swim Suit or Sports Bra to Labor In
- Socks/Slippers
- Breast Pads (In case your milk comes in early)
- Glasses (if needed)
- Books/Magazines
- Focus Item

For The Partner:

- The Birth Plan
- All Paperwork/Registration Information
- ID Cards
- Insurance Card
- Phone and charger
- Camera
- Ipod/Music Source
- Change of clothes
- Comfortable Shoes
- Cash (Small Bills)
- Ipad/Laptop
- Food/Snacks
- Water/Drinks
- Champagne (To take the edge off – or to celebrate afterward)

For The Baby:

- Diapers (Cloth or Disposable)
- Wipes (Cloth or Disposable)
- Onesies – Easy to wear, comfortable (key word) clothes for baby
- Baby Socks
- Take Home Outfit
- Blankets
- Baby Book for footprints
- Car Seat

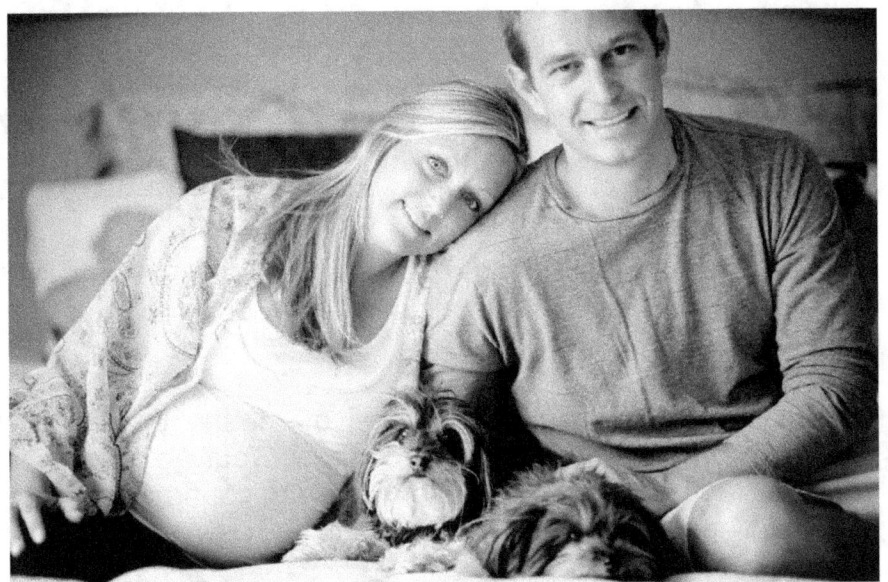

Chapter 23
The Partner's Role in the 3rd Trimester

Again, this chapter is written for the partner in the pregnancy. While every trimester of pregnancy is important, the final countdown can start to feel a bit overwhelming for you. I want to help you figure out the best way to support your partner through the third trimester, labor, and into parenthood.

I have many dads (and moms) come to me for care, and many of them ask questions about their partner's pregnancy. They, like you, want to be as supportive and helpful as possible.

The first thing you should know is that you are needed. No matter how independent and all-knowing your partner is, she needs you.

While the following are meant for you during pregnancy, please try to practice them throughout your relationship. Taking an active role in maintaining a strong connection is key to sustaining your bond.

Actively Communicate

Talk and listen. Truly hear her, and ask to be heard. You want to be on the same page, or at least understand the best you can what she is going through and what she would like for her birth. But you have a say too. Share what you want for this birth experience too. Opening up about your fears and hopes will help her to see that you are an active and invested support partner.

Become Educated about Birth

There are books that focus solely on you as the father throughout the pregnancy, and how you play an important role. As I have said, I highly recommend "Husband-Coached Childbirth." You want to skip the "What to Expect" series and others like it because they will not paint the proper picture of pregnancy and birth. You want to know what is happening and how to be there for her.

My co-author is a Bradley Childbirth instructor, and I highly recommend registering for the 12 week course. I know it is a time commitment, but I promise you it is worth it. When my clients take a birth series like this, it makes a difference in their labor experience. The class is not geared just to the mother, but to both of you.

Exercise Together

She is feeling tired and unmotivated right now, and as her coach, it is your job to help her stay active. Go for long walks together, swim, hit the gym, or take yoga. This is a bonding experience as well as a healthy lifestyle habit.

Eat Well

It is hard to reach for the right foods when you are craving something else entirely. While a midnight run for chocolate chip cookie dough is what she wants, try to keep both of your diets in check. Include over 75 grams of high quality protein a day and limit or eliminate processed foods. Read more about the Brewers Pregnancy Diet and all of the benefits it poses for her and your baby.

Practice Relaxation Together

The key to a natural labor is relaxation. Practicing emotional, physical, and mental relaxation during the third trimester will help prepare you both for the big day. There are many techniques to try: massage, reading, breathing rhythms, etc. Try practicing something each night with the goal being to relax her to sleep. Mentally note what techniques she enjoys and throw out the ones that made her laugh. One thing you can do is wake up in the middle of the night and look at her sleep position. This is the time she is in her most relaxed state. Help her try to mimic that position in the evenings when you work on relaxing.

De-Stress

Stress can cause issues with the baby and the pregnancy. Help out however you can so that she feels minimal amounts of it. It you have an argument, work it out. Any internally harbored feelings that aren't sorted through can disrupt labor and ruin a birth plan. This goes for stress over in-laws, friendships, fears, finances, work, etc. Speaking of finances, try to take the burden off of her going back to work immediately by taking over bills and money. Try to live off of your earnings and save to allow her the option of extending her maternity leave.

Go Play

If you have the chance to catch up with friends, or see a baseball game, do it. Invite your partner of course, but don't be disappointed if she would rather lay around. Your world is about to change in the best way possible, and your hobbies may slow down until you all get into a good flow at home. On that note, enjoy a few more date nights together too!

Plan Your Time Off

Talk to your place of work about taking time off for the birth and afterward. Ask for flexibility, as you will either leave when labor begins or call in if it begins at home. Talk to your partner about what she would like. I suggest spreading your days off out instead of taking them all at once!

Marinate over your childhood experiences and your parents' relationship

This is important. Look back on your relationship with your dad and pull from what you learned. What would you change? Also, look at the bond between your parents. How do you want your relationship to be with your partner? It takes effort to make these things last. Revisit these goals every so often to ensure that you constantly working toward the family life you want.

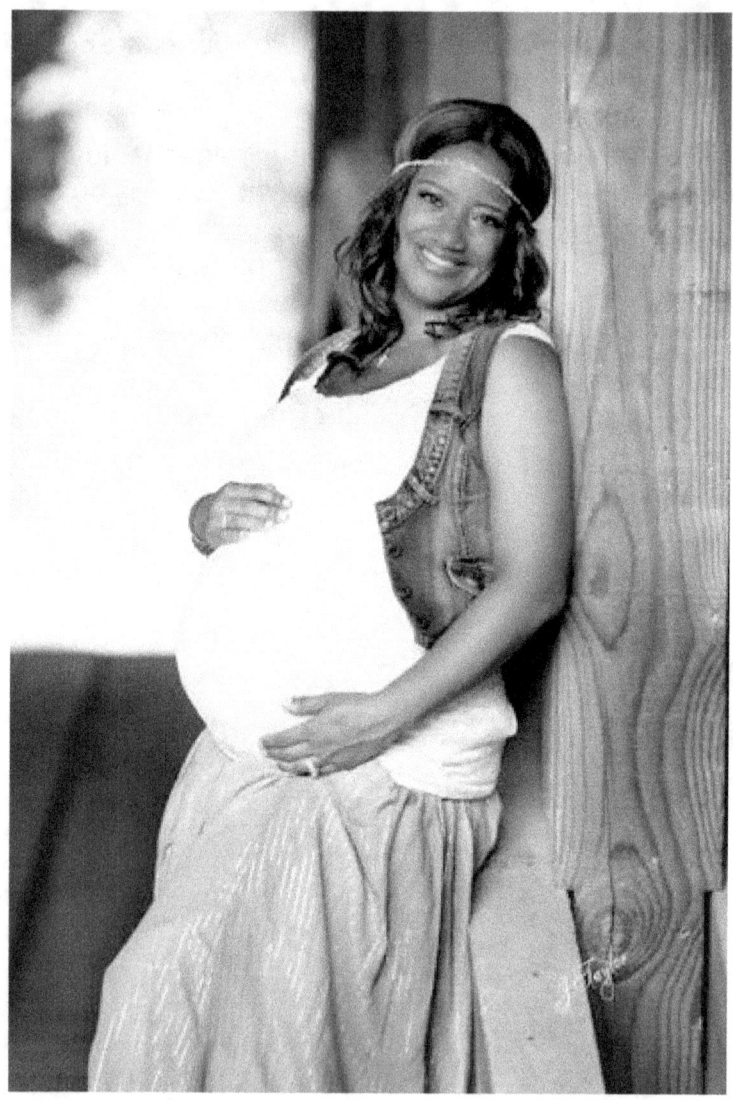

Chapter 24
3rd Trimester for Baby: Grow Baby Grow!

Welcome to the final countdown. You are so close to holding your baby.

The third trimester marks the final 12-14 weeks of growing in-utero for your baby. You may feel as though he has no more space to grow into inside of you, but somehow your body expands farther. While it is hard to be patient, it is well worth it. The longer your baby bakes, the healthier he should be once earth side.

So what is going on in there right now?

At this point in pregnancy, babies begin to develop on their own timeline. This means that what happens to one baby at week 30 may not occur until week 31 for your baby. This is one of the biggest reasons you should wait until you naturally go into labor instead of being induced. One baby may be ready at 38 weeks, while your baby needs 3 more weeks in the womb.

All organs and body parts are completely formed by the 28th week of pregnancy. (204) (205) (206) (207)

Weeks 28-30

- Healthy babies born around this time have a 90% chance of survival with medical help and without life-long effects.

- Baby can open their eyes, but it is too dark to see much inside the womb. They can differentiate between the brightness and the dark.
- They can hear you and recognize different sounds and voices.
- Starting to store fat on his body.
- All of his bones have formed, but they are still quite soft. With bone development comes bone marrow and red blood cell production.
- Practicing the grabbing motion by opening and closing his hands and sucking his thumb.
- Kicks and punches are quite strong and can take your breath away!
- The respiratory system is still maturing and now produces surfactant, which helps the lungs fill with air.
- The nervous system is still developing but can control some body functions
- Baby may weigh around 3lbs now.

Weeks 31-34

- Lungs are not yet fully developed, and need more time before they breath 'outside' air, but there are rhythmic breathing movements taking place as they practice for coming earth side.
- The fine lanugo hair is starting to disappear and the skin is becoming more pink and less opaque. Some babies hold on to their peach-fuzz hair until a few weeks after birth, so don't be alarmed if your baby has hair on their back or ears!
- Your baby will be descending into birthing position, hopefully head down.
- Eyesight is becoming more developed.
- Iron and calcium are being stored, along with fat.
- All the fat that is being stored is helping with brain growth, as well as body fat growth.

Weeks 35-38

- Your baby's nervous system can now control his body temperature.
- Movements are felt as he stretches and rolls, but remains low in the pelvis and engaged for birth.
- Lungs are still 'practicing' and are not yet completely ready. Once they are fully mature (generally between 38-40 weeks, but there are always exceptions), a chemical is released that alters the mother's hormones.
- Small breast buds are forming. They will feel hard to the touch and be locate under his nipples, but will soften during the first few weeks of life.
- Your little baby is packing on the weight now. They will gain an average of ½ pound a week from now until birth.
- Baby is getting antibodies from you that will help protect him from illnesses after birth.
- At 37 weeks, he is considered 'Early-Term.' This means that if he decides to come on his own, everything should be just fine, but he is not yet at the 39 week 'Full-Term' mark.

Weeks 39-42

- Your baby has made it to 'Full Term.'
- Your baby's movements lessen as the womb is becoming crowded and labor is around the corner, but kick counts can still be done to keep Mom calm.
- Head may be rapidly growing hair (or they could be a bald baby!).
- Nails are all growing, and will probably need clipped soon after birth.
- The vernix that once covered him, thick and white, is falling off in the womb. The longer he bakes, the less you will see on his skin at birth. (Don't forget to rub that

natural lotion into baby's skin after birth, it helps with the seeding process and is quite beneficial.)

- Your baby's brain is soaking up the healthy fats and so is his body.
- The bones to the skull are still soft. They will remain soft so they can mold and move for the birth process to take place.
- Baby will weigh between 6-9lbs on average at birth, depending on when birth occurs, with the average length being 19-21 inches.
- Birth will happen when baby is ready, but typically occurs within this window of time.

Chapter 25
Breech Babies

You are well into the third trimester, and your OB or midwife has identified your baby as being in the breech position.

Now what? They say, "Give it time! The baby will turn on his own!" But what if they don't? You can be more proactive in helping your baby get into a better position. The sooner the baby is in optimal position, the better the brain and spinal development of the baby will be.

When you learn that your baby is not in typical birthing position, you may hear one of the following terms:

Frank Breech: This means your baby's bottom is down first with his legs up by his head.

Footling or Incomplete Breech: Your baby has one or both feet downward.

Complete Breech: Your baby is cross legged.

Babies can also be **transverse**, which means the baby is laying sideways. This typically occurs more with 2nd pregnancies.

They may also be in a posterior position, which usually means you will have a lot of back pain and back labor.

Complete breech   Frank breech   Incomplete breech

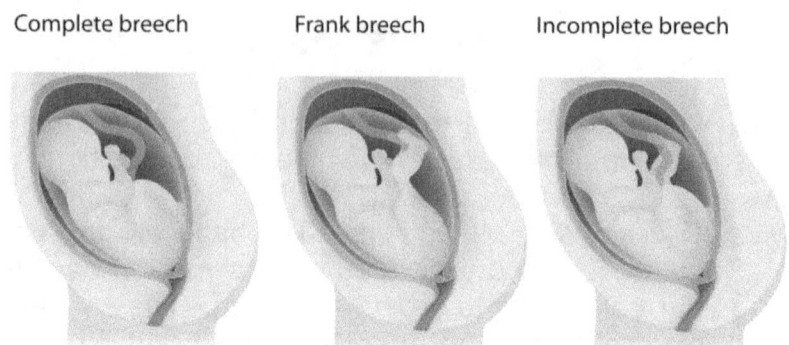

What are some things you can do to help get baby in better position?

Chiropractic care should be first and foremost. Make sure the chiropractor is certified in the Webster Technique like I have discussed previously. Balancing the maternal pelvis to help the muscles and ligaments relax will help with baby moving into optimal position. (209)

Acupuncture is considered a form of Chinese medicine that helps to balance the meridians and allow the chi(energy) to flow freely. Small needles are inserted in the skin at specific points the provider has determined will help restore the energy flow. We see a lot of success when chiropractic and acupuncture are used together.

Moxibustion technique is used by many acupuncturists. It is also designed to improve the chi flow. This is a form of heat therapy in which mugwort(herb) is burned near the surface of the skin. It is a great alternative if you do not like needles. Talk to your acupuncturist to see which is best for you.

Other options:

- Talk to your baby. Read to him. Stimulate him.

- Babies do not like the cold. You can put an ice pack over his head with a heating pad over the pubic bone to try to turn your baby. You can also use a flashlight or some music down near the groin to help encourage him to move into a better position.

- I like to use an oil blend of peppermint and myrrh. Mix 3-5 drops of each with a teaspoon of coconut oil and rub on the belly in the direction to encourage the baby to go head down. The peppermint has a cooling effect while the myrrh has a warming feeling.

- Red Raspberry leaf tea which natural has magnesium, potassium, and vitamin C is wonderful to be taking during pregnancy. Depending where you are in your pregnancy depends how much you drink. There are all different reports of when and how much tea you should be drinking. I usually have my mom start drinking in the first trimester.
½ cup – one cup a day. Then 2 cups in 2nd trimester and 3 cups in the third. Red raspberry is great for uterine and fertility health, helps to relax the uterus if baby is in a breech position. The tea can also help with leg cramps and some moms to be say they sleep better too. You can buy in the store, or we carry tea from our local herbalist in the office.

- One of my favorite websites to go to for all things breech is www.spinningbabies.com. I know that I mentioned the site earlier, but it really is worth looking at. There is plenty of information there to help your little one get into a better position. I have taken the class myself and found it very helpful.

- Hamstring stretches. Great for loosening up the pelvis and glute muscles. Put your foot up on a stool or chair and bend forward. You should only feel a stretch in the hamstring and not the back. I prefer this way to stretch, as it saves your back during pregnancy and not putting extra strain on your back.

- Cat/Cow yoga poses. I like to have my mom's do this several times a day. If you do not have time, at least do it before bed. As many babies like to find their head down in the middle of the night when you are the most relaxed. These poses help to not only relax the back muscles, helps to open up the pelvis and its muscles, and stretches the round and broad ligaments of the uterus. Can also help with "back labor" pains and hip pain as well.
- Relax! Keep your stress level low. Meditate, color, think happy thoughts all to help lower stress and maintain cortisol levels.
- Hit the pool. Helps to relax both you and baby. If you can, doing somersaults in the water can help. As well as rolling like a log. Swimming helps take gravity off your body, so both you and your baby are weightless.

As you can see, there are plenty of things you can do to help get your baby into better position. Most of my mom's do not feel the baby move into position, most of the time it happens in the middle of the night. Some moms have told me it was uncomfortable when the baby moved if they were standing, some had a lot of back pain or sciatica as the baby was getting into position. Those are rare, but I just wanted you to be aware of what you might feel.

Chapter 26
Group B Strep: Make an Informed Decision

GBS is so common within pregnancy conversations that it has become a running laughable topic. It seems that every pregnant woman you meet talks about having to be given IV antibiotics during labor due to GBS. As if it is just part of the protocol. But why? And is it really necessary?

What is Group B Strep?

Group B Strep is *NORMAL*. Let me repeat, NORMAL. It is a *normal* bacteria found in the gut.

If it is normal, why are we made to believe that it is so scary to have? Even deadly? The problem is thought to be when these bacteria multiply during pregnancy and become a danger to your health and potentially to your baby's health. GBS will not kill your baby unless it goes completely undetected and untreated, which would be pretty rare.

Most newborns born with GBS will make a full recovery, but if it is not treated, it can cause life-threatening complications, such as: (210)

- blood poisoning (septicaemia)
- pneumonia
- meningitis

Your doctor will perform the Group B Strep Test sometime during weeks 35-37. Some midwives offer the test as optional now – which is a huge step forward. If you decide to get the test done, I would recommend doing it as early as they allow so you can get your results quickly. Positive results (again, these results do not mean that you will pass the bacteria to your baby) read early give you time to reduce the bacteria and take another test. That way you won't have to refuse the antibiotics at birth. Remember though that on any given day you can test positive or negative because the bacteria are always present, it just depends on the amount on the day you are tested. So performing preventative measures or treatment protocol can be done, and then you should ask for another test to be done.

I feel like I need to repeat this: A positive test result does not mean that you have the GBS disease or that your baby will become ill.(211) Your doctor will, however, tell you that antibiotics are absolutely necessary while you are in labor – often several rounds of them. If you test positive, you can opt for these antibiotics, but remember just how antibiotics effect your gut health – and the gut of your baby. There are other options.

Based on the fact that we aren't even sure that the antibiotic typically given at birth actually prevents GBS from passing to the baby, over 50,000 women are treated to prevent 1 neonatal death – again, that's if the antibiotics are capable of preventing this. (212) Remember too that GBS signs typically arise within the first hours after birth and can be treated at that point.   But you can watch for signs for up to 6 weeks after birth.

Signs of GBS in your newborn include: (213)

- Anxious or stressed appearance

- Blue appearance (cyanosis)

- Breathing difficulties, such as flaring of the nostrils, grunting noises, rapid breathing, and short periods without breathing

- Irregular or abnormal heart rate, they may be fast or very slow

- Lethargy

- Pale appearance (pallor) with cold skin

- Poor feeding

- Unstable body temperature (low or high)

The following are found too increase your newborn's risk of contracting GBS: (213)(214)

- Preterm Labor and Premature Birth (prior to 37 weeks)

- Mother who has already given birth to a baby with GBS sepsis

- Mother who has a fever of 100.4°F (38°C) or higher during labor

- Mother who has group B streptococcus in her gastrointestinal, reproductive, or urinary tract

- Rupture of membranes (water breaks) more than 18 hours before the baby is delivered

- Use of intrauterine fetal monitoring (scalp lead) during labor

According to the Cochrane Database, "There is lack of

evidence from well designed and conducted trials to recommend Intrapartum antibiotic prophylaxis to reduce neonatal GBS." (338)

Did You Know?

Bacteria is passed to your baby before he is born, helping to create the foundation of his own gut bacteria. This would mean that GBS is contracted prior to birth, and instead while the baby is still in the womb. Are you following me on this? This leads us to believe then that the antibiotics given at birth are useless. If your baby contracted GBS in utero already, the antibiotics will not change that.

There is no way to know if your baby contracted GBS until after he is born and shows signs of the illness. So treating preemptively can cause more harm than good.
Our society is famous for treating pregnancies 'on a conveyor belt.' It is time to start treating each woman as an individual. Watching for signs of GBS after birth allow for far fewer women and infants to be exposed to unnecessary antibiotics and side effects.

If you have had any yeast infections during your pregnancy, it is a sign that your good bacteria in your gut is becoming out numbered.

The following are possible ways to avoid testing positive for GBS:

- A diet void of excess sugar
- Avoid antibiotics and medications during pregnancy
- Increase your probiotic dosage for at least two weeks before your scheduled test
- Consume ample garlic orally and consider inserting a clove vaginally at night for a week or two before the test

day. Garlic is a natural antibiotic and bacteria cannot live in the presence of it.

If you test positive and want to treat naturally, consider the following:

A natural treatment will help to restore healthy vaginal bacteria.

- **High potency probiotic supplement**: This can be taken orally or vaginally. Intake at least 4 billion cells per dose. You can use an organic tampon and roll it in coconut oil and then the probiotic and insert it for several hours. This will help with GBS as well as and yeast that may me hiding as well! Don't forget to eat probiotic-rich foods too. Coconut Oil also has antiviral properties, so enjoy some daily.

- **Garlic**: Oral and Vaginally.
- **Vitamin C**
- **Burdock Root and Echinacea Root Infusion**
- **Echinacea and Astragalus Tinctures**
- **Grapefruit Seed Extract**

Did You Know?

It is so important to remember that there is healthy bacteria your baby will receive as he passes through the birth canal. Taking the antibiotics recommended while you are in labor will prevent your baby from receiving ALL of these bacteria. *This alters his immune system and can place his gut at risk.* With the good bacteria eliminated, you and your baby have little to no defense system in place to prevent new germs, bacteria, and viruses from invading your bodies while you are in the hospital. (The hospital is FULL of germs.) Antibiotics also lead to the problems of 'super bugs' (antibiotic resistant) which are resistant to normal strength antibiotics. It is also widely known now just how closely the gut health is linked to autism symptoms. Keep all of this in mind before agreeing to any vaccinations as well, as they can alter the gut bacteria.

It has been shown that babies who receive antibiotics at birth or shortly after birth have less diversity of their gut bacteria at 4 and 8 weeks after their antibiotic treatment. This leaves them at higher risk for illnesses, chronic problems, and conditions such as yeast growth (thrush). (215)

Antibiotics should only be used if absolutely necessary – and when all other methods of correcting a bacterial imbalance have been completely exhausted.

PART 3

Labor

Preparing and educating yourself for the birth you want.

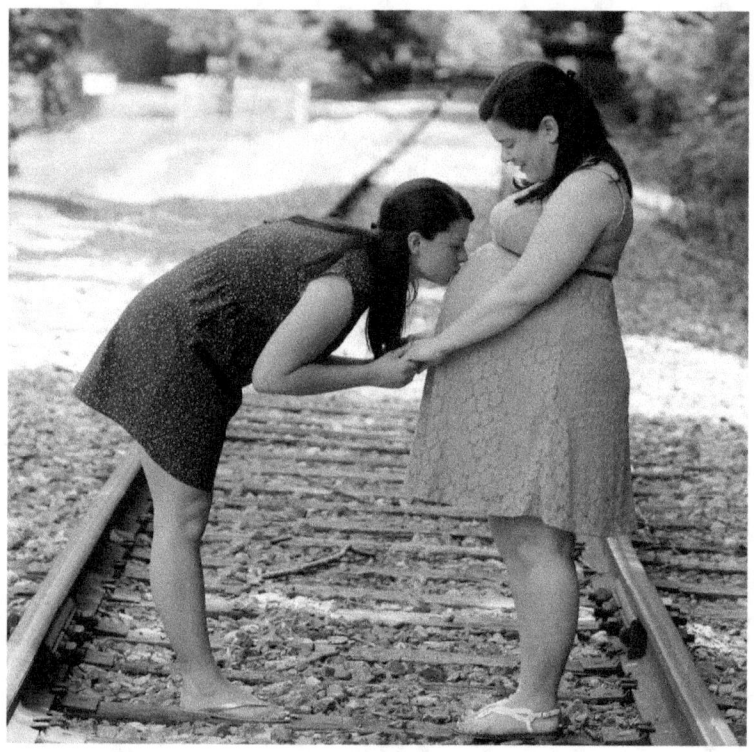

"At some point during labor, you will feel as though you truly cannot do it. That is when your baby is coming." – unkown.

Chapter 27
Preparing For Labor

Did you know that most couples spend more time working on their baby registry than they do preparing for labor? They spend more time dreaming and setting up a nursery than educating themselves on birthing.

Do not fall into this category! Do not just walk into the two-hour hospital class that covers a medicated birth, bathing/swaddling, and breastfeeding basics all in one breath. You only have one shot at this pregnancy, this birth, and this baby's infancy. You will make plenty of mistakes, but you want to have no regrets.
Whether this is your first birth or your fourth, take the time to educate yourself.

I want to start by saying that your partner should be prepared too. This will not only help YOU through labor, but it will bring the two of you closer than you thought you could be. There are other wonderful books out there on birthing, and I highly recommend that you read as many as you can! Even if you don't plan a natural, unmedicated birth, read like you are because you will learn more about the body and its capabilities.

There is no "normal" when it comes to labor. Doctors like to tell you that the average woman dilates at a centimeter an hour and then pushes for two hours. This is based on the curve of all women, meaning that very few are actually in this category and most fall on either side. I have watched couples labor for 70 hours (HEROES) and couples wake up with contractions 2 minutes apart and hold a baby within 2 hours (EQUALLY HEROES – hello downhill part of a rollercoaster!!). The truth is that your labor is designed to birth your baby. No one can predict how fast or slow it will go. Being prepared for the crazy intensity of either side of the bell curve is key to being mentally ready to birth.

Throughout this section of the book, you are going to read about birth in all of its glory. Each chapter is dedicated toward aiding you in reaching your own personal goals of labor; and by the end, you will be able to create a birth plan with your true priorities in mind.

"You are constructing your own reality with the choices you make ... or don't make. If you really want a healthy pregnancy and joyful birth, and you truly understand that you are the one in control, then you must examine what you have or haven't done so far to create the outcome you want."

-Kim Wildner

Chapter 28
Relaxation, the Key to a Natural Labor

Every woman handles stress and pain differently. Do you yell? Curse? Cry? Sleep? Need a hug? Want to be alone?

These are important things to know about yourself, as they may play a rather large part in your labor. Learning your instincts will help you find the best methods of relaxation, and as you are about to learn, relaxation is the key to a successful unmedicated birth.

Even if you plan on receiving medical interventions such as epidurals and Pitocin, you need to know that there's a chance the medicine won't work for you, will wear off before the end of labor, will cause major side effects, or just plain doesn't get to you in time.

Practicing your relaxation techniques throughout your pregnancy will reduce your stress levels, which you know is important, and increase the chances of a successful natural birth.

Before you start laughing at some of the following techniques, remember just how different everyone is; what works for one woman may not for another. Try them all and find a few that will benefit you.

Why You Need To Practice Relaxing

Labor can be compared to a marathon. You wouldn't show up and attempt to run (and finish) a marathon on the day of the race, right? So don't show up unprepared for your labor!

Your body works better when it is relaxed. Practicing different relaxation techniques throughout your pregnancy will allow them to occur more naturally during labor. The hormones that aid in progressing labor will be released easier if you are relaxed. And letting the body give in to the labor by relaxing allows the body to store energy and possibly aids baby in coping and adapting to the birth experience.

Oxytocin is a hormone released when you are in love, in labor, or are breastfeeding; it is what makes you feel loopy and not quite present. Relaxing will allow your body to soak up this oxytocin better during labor. Did you know that some women even claim they can orgasm during this experience? That would take extreme relaxation and the ability to completely let go. If an orgasm is not on your birth plan, but you are hoping to have the most peaceful experience possible, that too takes relaxation. So please consider this chapter your daily homework from now until your baby arrives.

Always utilize abdominal breathing during relaxation practice, and have your partner remind you to do so during labor as well. Make sure that your breaths come from your belly and not your chest; shallow breaths will trigger stress and anxiety, creating the cycle of fear, and can lead to hyper-ventilating.

The average contraction is 60 seconds in length, so practicing your techniques for 60 seconds at a time should be your goal. Your relaxation practice should include the following:

- While laying down, let yourself completely relax. This means your limbs and fingers/toes are not moving, your head becomes heavy with your eyes closing, even

189

your mouth falls slightly open. Let your mind drift away to a place that makes you feel comfort and happiness.

- While sitting, let the limbs and head 'dangle' and focus on your breath. Inhale for a count of 4-5 and exhale for a count of 8-10. Make it rhythmic.
- While standing, lean against a wall or forward over a chair or table, and imagine a warm gentle waterfall rolling over you – beginning at your head and covering each inch of you. Focus on nothing else but the warming sensation.
- Use music as a way to let your mind drift away.
- Dance, rock back and forth slowly while standing or on your hands and knees, hug over your birthing ball, or sway in the shower. A swaying motion tends to be very relaxing.
- Have your support partner massage you. A back rub, foot rub, or hand massage may help you release tension. There are many techniques you can practice to find a few that you really enjoy.
- Rebozoing is the act of removing the weight and pain from the birthing mother by using a rebozo (a large piece of fabric) to lift the belly and sway it gently while the mother is on her hands and knees.

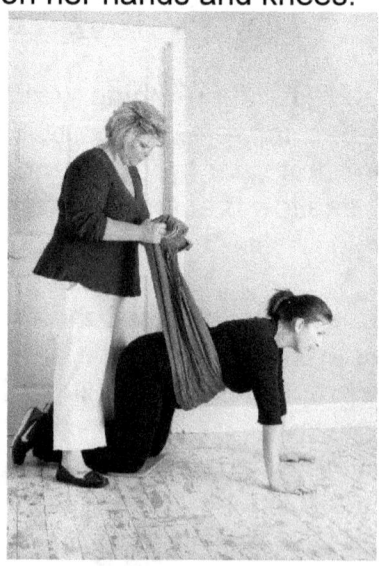

- Self-hypnosis can be obtained by total relaxation.
- Rhythmic/Ocean Breathing: Breathing in rhythm to the ocean is my personal favorite way to handle contractions. Inhale as if you are the wave returning to the ocean and
exhale as it crashes to the sand.
- Floating: You've had the warm water feeling flow over you through the waterfall relaxation. Now imagine as if you're floating on water. Let the water sway you back and forth and rock you to sleep.
- Sleeping: The ultimate form of relaxation is sleep.
- Guided Imagery: Repeating, and seeing, the colors of the rainbow, mentally visiting a special place, listening to a story read aloud, these are all methods of visually creating relaxation.

Try following these visualization steps:
- Think of an experience you've had that was entirely stress-free, an enjoyable moment of calmness and contentment.
- Think of where this event happened and picture it in your mind.
- Imagine the sounds, tastes, smells, and feelings.
- Stay in the moment as if time no longer matters, but place your current self in the image – pregnant and beautiful.
- Let the waves of contractions come and go peacefully while you are in this place of happiness.

Another great wat to achieve relaxation is by adding birth affirmations to your practice (and labor). Repeating an affirmation has the power to relax the mind and body. You can create your own affirmation or pick a few from this list:

- My baby will come in his way, on his own timeline.
- I trust my body to birth my baby.
- My body is strong enough to birth this baby.
- I am strong and capable.
- There is peace within me.

- Give in and let go.
- This is my baby's journey, and I am his guide.
- I will let the waves wash over me.
- I am a mother, and I will comfort and love this baby.
- Every contraction brings me closer to my baby.
- The stronger my contractions become, the sooner I meet my baby.
- I breathe slowly and easily, and it helps my body let go.
- My breath is felt by my baby.
- I open my body to birth my baby.
- I am calm, I am loved, I am relaxed.
- My labor cannot be stronger than I am.
- I control the pain; I control the peace.
- Each contraction comes from me. Each contraction is meant for my baby.
- I will let my baby guide this birth.

Make sure that you create a relaxing environment to practice in. This 'safe haven' will be your comfort zone when active labor progresses. I recommend staying at home for as long as possible before moving to a sterile hospital environment – or different environment in general, as a change of locations can stall or halt labor all together.

If you need to be at your birth place in early labor, then bring things that will allow the environment to be as relaxing as possible for you. (Flameless candles, music, pillows, essential oils, etc)

Remember that practicing daily will bring you confidence as your labor begins. You will naturally fall into your relaxation as your labor progresses, and you will feel more capable and empowered as you bring your baby earth side.

Chapter 29
What You Should Know About Epidurals

Epidurals are given very frequently across our nation, but never fully discussed within our society. Over ¾ of vaginal deliveries occur with an epidural. I personally had an "emergency c-section" and I was never once told about the side effects or any of the possibilities of what could happen. I just want to make sure you have the information to make an informed choice.

Because epidurals are given so often then it must mean it is a safe choice, right?

WRONG.

The first recorded use of an epidural was in 1885, when a New York neurologist injected *cocaine* into the back of a patient . Over a century later, epidurals have become the most popular method of pain relief during labor.

The research is overwhelming – as in 'WHY is this drug cocktail being shot into the backs of laboring women VOLUNTARILY?' It is because we don't know better. It is true, this is your decision to make. I do not judge, but I do educate. I'm going to lay it all out there, and then you will be able to make the best decision for you.

There is still much we don't understand about birth, and even more we don't have direct control over. Despite a woman's best efforts to have a natural, undisturbed birth, complications can occur that require medical attention. *In these circumstances, whatever interventions may protect the health and safety of both the mother and baby are what should take place. At the end of the day, that is by far more important than how the baby was born.*

What is an Epidural?

I want to start with the basics; understanding the different types of epidurals, how they are administered, and their benefits and risks will help you in your decision-making during the course of labor and delivery.(216)

The Epidural: The anesthesiologist will insert a needle between the tough, outer membrane that covers the spinal cord and the membrane just below that. A catheter is threaded through the needle and left in place after the needle is removed to administer the medication as needed. An anesthetic, typically a mixture of anesthetic and narcotic, is injected into the catheter. There are two ways in which the epidural medication is administered:

Continuous Infusion: This is when a pump gradually delivers a continuous dose through a syringe attached to the catheter. This tends to be the most common choice, as it provides steady labor pain relief.

Intermittent Top-Ups: This is when the anesthesiologist returns to inject more pain medication into the catheter when the dose wears off.

The "Walking" or "Light" Epidural: The anesthesiologist may inject narcotic only, or a very low dose of anesthetic, or a combination of the two in an attempt to achieve pain relief with mobility. These variations are intended to leave some sensation and ability to move the legs. This is still a huge interference with your labor, as many women with such epidurals never walk, even when encouraged to do so.

The Combined Spinal-Epidural: This is when the anesthesiologist injects the pain medication into the space that lies deeper than the epidural space (known as a "spinal"). The anesthesiologist then pulls outward into the epidural space, threads a catheter into the epidural space, and removes the needle. The spinal cannot be repeated, but the catheter remains for an epidural should you want additional labor pain relief later. (217)

Novocain is commonly used as a spinal anesthesia, but according to the warnings about Novocain, it may cause adverse fetal development, and is not recommended for pregnant women. It may cause severe hypertension with the possibility of rupturing a cerebral blood vessel. (218)

Epidural medications fall into a class of drugs called local anesthetics, and are often combined with opioids or narcotics in order to decrease the required dose of local anesthetic during labor.

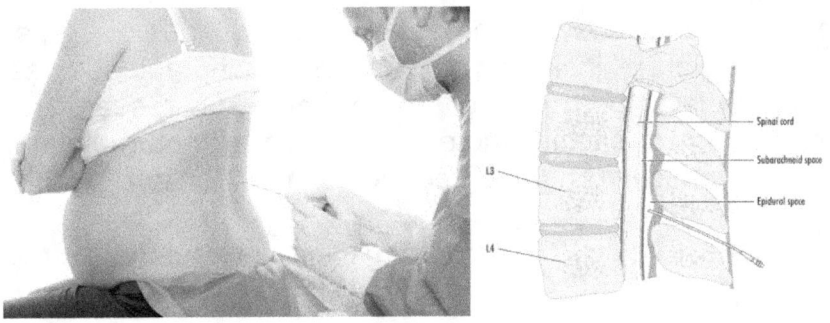

If you choose an epidural, you will be asked to curl up on your side or sit up with your back arched outward. Your back will be washed with antiseptic and covered with a sterile drape. The anesthesiologist will numb the skin before inserting the needle. You must remain absolutely still while the needle is in your back.

Did You Know?

With an epidural comes:

- An IV: About a quart of IV fluid is administered before the epidural is given.

- Frequent monitoring of mom and baby (continuous EFM)

Getting an epidural increases the need for Pitocin by 3 fold. The combination of epidurals and Pitocin, drastically increase the chances of needing instrumental help with the delivery of your baby. Both of these medications cause abnormal fetal heart rate changes that can be linked to fetal distress.

Pitocin is a synthetic oxytocin. In 2012, a study was conducted by *Australian and New Zealand Journal of Gynecology* that showed the use of Pitocin leads to "great pain and suffering, including serious unintended and adverse health effects to both mother and infant." The researchers concluded that pitocin increased "severe maternal and neonatal morbidity" and doubled the risk of c-section. (219)

Pitocin Side Effects (directly from the manufacturer's drug insert):

- Anaphylactic reaction
- Postpartum hemorrhage
- Cardiac arrhythmia
- Fatal afibrinogenemia
- Nausea
- Vomiting
- Premature ventricular contractions
- Pelvic hematoma
- Subarachnoid hemorrhage
- Hypertensive episodes
- Rupture of the uterus

According to the same drug insert, the infant may suffer due to the intensity of the contractions. This can lead to:

- Bradycardia
- Premature ventricular contractions and other arrhythmias
- Permanent CNS or brain damage
- Fetal death
- Neonatal seizures have been reported

Not only are you at a higher risk of receiving Pitocin with an epidural, but you are also more likely to receive:

- drugs to fight a drop in blood pressure

- a urinary catheter for inability to pass urine

- a vacuum extraction or a forceps delivery.

- cesarean section. (220)

I have seen many mothers who have dealt with injuries from their epidurals. Not only from the epidural itself, but at the site of the injection. I also see several fractured tailbones, sacrums, and hips from the fact moms cannot feel or tell their bones are breaking.

An epidural may cause (221)

- Fever in labor, which is linked to infants needing blood draws for possible infection, and even resuscitation at birth: A recent study found that epidural-related fevers can lead to problems including poor muscle tone, difficulty breathing, seizures and low Apgar scores. (222)

- A severe headache caused by leakage of spinal fluid.

- A stalled or slowed labor
- Ringing of the ears
- Shivering
- Chronic backache
- Nausea
- Difficulty urinating.
- Numbness.
- Permanent nerve damage
- serious tears in your perineum

- adverse behavioral effects for your baby

- newborn jaundice

- life-threatening complications (dangerously low blood pressure, respiratory or cardiac arrest, severe allergic reaction, convulsion)

First-time mothers tend to have more difficulties with epidural side effects than women who have previously given birth.

20% of women who receive an epidural end up with an unplanned c-section. (220)

Did You Know?

Having an epidural while in labor can negatively affect your breastfeeding relationship. Mothers who receive an epidural have more difficulty in the first week, and are more likely to give up breastfeeding within the first six months. Research shows that the intervention can interfere with a baby's ability to correctly suck at the breast. (223)(224)

The epidural also enters the baby's bloodstream through the placenta and umbilical cord, which has a large impact on the placenta, causing it to block oxidized stresses and other processes that are supposed to take place during labor. The medication can also make it difficult for some babies to get into a good birth position. (225)

"The whole point of woman-centered birth is the knowledge that a woman is the birth power source. She may need, and deserve, help, but in essence, she always had, currently has, and will have the power." -Heather McCue

Chapter 30

Family-Centered C-Sections

In 2014, over 32% of birthing women had a cesarean section.(226) This statistic is at a scary level in our country, which ironically also has an increasing number of maternal deaths during childbirth each year as well as a rising intervention to labor rate. (227) The World Health Organization has stated numerous times that these numbers must come down. Most recently, they have acknowledged that medical inductions increase the chances of 'emergency c-sections' occurring, and they have raised the full-term label from 37 weeks to 39 weeks with the hope that less inductions will occur. (228)

Obviously, you should avoid a c-section at all costs, but there are times when the surgery is absolutely necessary and life-saving for mother or baby. For some women with pre-existing conditions, a c-section actually allows them the ability to carry a pregnancy and give birth.

I have worked with women who did end up on the operating table, and by understanding their options and knowing how to handle the surgery, they still had very happy births! I have also worked with women who knew they would have a c-section due to health complications or prior birth issues. They all truly wanted a peaceful, calm, loving birth environment -- and they got it. When you are educated on all of your rights – even during a c-section – you can still have a peaceful birth!

A cesarean section is a surgical procedure used to deliver a baby through incisions in the mother's abdomen *and* uterus. Please watch actual c-section videos (online) so that you have a better understanding of what takes place during the surgery.

You need to watch to really know that it is an abdominal surgery and it will take time to recover afterward. You want to watch to know exactly what is happening to your body so that you can discuss with your surgical team your desires and hopes.

If you find yourself in need of a c-section, you do not have to lie back and give up on your birth. Many women are opting for a gentle cesarean, a family-centered surgical birth. This allows for you to feel involved in your birth, lowers the risk of a traumatic birth experience for you, and provides a stronger foundation for initial bonding, increasing your chances of successful breastfeeding and lowering chances of postpartum depression.

What is a gentle, family-centered c-section?

In a typical c-section, a closed curtain shields the family from witnessing the surgery. Mothers don't see the procedure and, typically, their babies are immediately whisked away for care.

Family-centered cesareans are new in the U.S., and many doctors and hospitals have no experience with them.

'Family-Centered' means exactly that: *The family is the focus of the surgical experience.*

From Family Centered Cesarean: (229)
"While there are very specific pieces that contribute to the family centered Cesarean, such as the lowering of the drape or lack of routine family separation in the immediate postpartum, the core of this practice remains the same as that of all client centered healthcare. The family is the focus. The family's needs and desires are heard by the medical staff who then makes every effort to ensure that these preferences are met. The staff that provides family centered Cesarean understands that every birth is a momentous occasion, and that the need for a baby to be born surgically does not negate

the need for the family to celebrate this wondrous time."

You may request a gentle cesarean for your birth, but your doctor may not be experienced with it. It is very important that you take the time to research exactly what you want and present it to your birth team. Create a birth plan for your surgery and cover it in depth with your doctor, reviewing it again just before the surgery is to take place. You have every right as a woman giving birth vaginally does to request and push for the birth that you want.

The gentle C-section is not a replacement for a vaginal birth; it's just a way to improve the surgical experience.

A doctor may see a gentle c-section as a bunch of little adjustments, but it can be so much more than this. Before creating your birth plan, talk to your doctor about every step of the surgical experience. You want to know what typically happens from the moment you enter the hospital and are admitted until you are wheeled out. It is very important that you know all of this in advance so you are not surprised by anything the day of your birth.

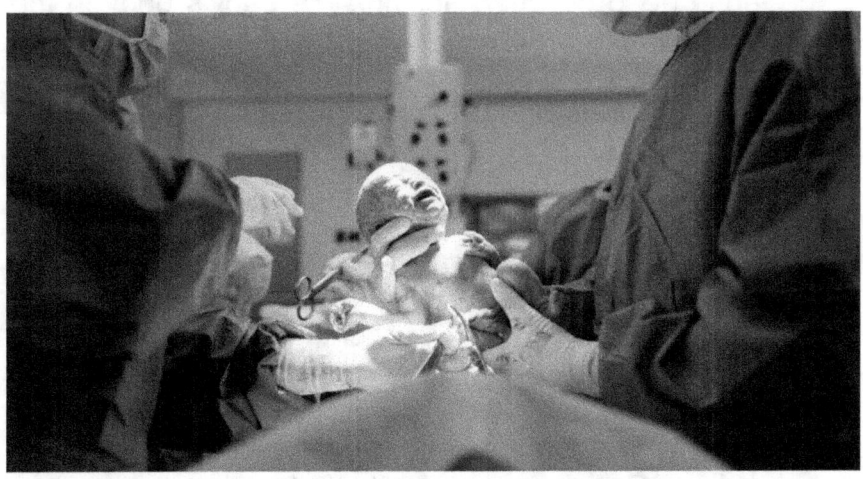

I've compiled a list of things to consider when creating your gentle, family-centered cesarean birth plan: (230)

1. Spouse, midwife and/or doula will be present
2. Gentle surgical techniques that end thin the least amount of cutting and scar tissue
3. The doctor will explain the surgery to out loud as it happens
4. Operating room conversation will be about my birth (not the doctor's weekend plans)
5. All medications are suitable for breastfeeding
6. No sedatives after birth
7. The uterus will be reinforced (to carry future- children)
8. Use dissolvable stitches for closing
9. Keep the dominant arm free for immediate contact with the newborn
10. Place blood pressure cuff on the non-dominant arm
11. Place the echocardiogram leads on the back or far laterally to facilitate early chest contact between mother and baby
12. Breastfeeding while happen in the OR
13. No oxygen mask
14. Clear drapes to view the birth (Or lower the drapes as aby is delivered)
15. Gentle head delivery, leaving the baby's body in the uterus for a few moments allowing one last contraction to help with breathing and clearing fluid from the lungs.

16. Delay cord clamping: (yes you can do this with a c-section!)

17. Any and all newborn exams done while mother's chest, or they should be delayed until after the baby has successfully latched and nursed

18. Mother and baby are not to be separated (even when leaving OR, you can cradle the baby on your chest)

19. Blankets available for warmth
20. Bring your own music into the operating room.
21. Request to eat and have the IV removed as soon as possible after surgery
22. Inquire about having a photographer in the operating room
23. Once in recovery, ask to be alone with your partner and baby for at least an hour for bonding time.
24. Be up and walking as soon as possible
25. Delay the first bath (until you are home)

In addition to these considerations, also include the following procedures or experiences to ensure the healthiest outcome:

Vaginal Seeding: You will read more about this in the next chapter, but early studies show that swabbing a mother's vagina and transferring it to her baby's mouth, eyes, and skin immediately following surgery may transfer bacteria similar to babies being born vaginally. Seeding may even protect from health issues later in life. (231) (232)

Immediate Skin-to-Skin: Having a c-section delays the initiation of breastfeeding, reduces the chances of an exclusive breastfeeding relationship, significantly delays the milk from 'coming in' and increases the likelihood of supplementing with formula. But by having immediate skin-to-skin following a cesarean, you increases the chances of a successful breastfeeding relationship! (233) (234)

Did You Know?

As long as you and baby are healthy after surgery, you can be taken to recovery together. You can practice skin-to-skin and breastfeed as often as possible with a lactation consultant, if needed. This time will help strengthen your bond and heal your emotional scars.

Make sure you rest at home, as the surgery is not a minor event. You will be offered medications, it is up to you to accept them. Do your research and hear your body.
You will need to heal emotionally. Reach out to support groups; write your story; grieve the birth you lost and find peace in the one you had. Please join the ICAN network.
http://www.ican-online.org/

Chapter 31
Vaginal Seeding

In the last chapter, you learned about having a beautiful c-section birth. Part of that experience may be the seeding of your baby. Research now shows us that babies born by c-section are linked to increased rates of obesity, asthma, celiac disease, autism, chronic illnesses, and type 1 diabetes later in their lives. (231) This research suggests that it is the differences in the bacteria of the gut that plays a role in this link to diseases. While many factors come in to play with these illnesses, it is quite remarkable that all recent research shares a common factor: the gut, and the gut bacteria.

Allowing the body to labor on its own, without intervention, provides a plethora of positives for both mom and baby, but allowing baby to pass through the birth canal has to take the cake! Our bodies are so amazing that we not only grow humans, but our own gut flora is passed to those humans as they grow, through the placenta. It gets even better; our gut bacteria travels from our gut into the birth canal during labor. These bacteria then are absorbed through baby's skin, eyes, nose, mouth, genitals, etc as he passes through the birth canal and is welcomed to the world. (235)

By having these bacteria absorbed into their bodies, babies have a decreased risk of the above mentioned illnesses, as well as many more.

If you are HIV negative, and having a C-Section, I highly recommend you seed your baby. If you are GBS positive, talk to your doctor about vaginal seeding. Most doctors will say that you will pass it to baby, but remember that only one in every 4,000 positive GBS women passes it to her child during birth. The odds of the other life-long chronic illnesses are much higher than that. Personally, I would still seed my child if I tested positive for GBS.

Dr. Maria Gloria Dominguez-Bello, an associate professor in the Human Microbiome Program at the NYU School of Medicine, defines the process of "seeding" a newborn as follows:

1. Take a piece of gauze soaked in saline
2. Fold it up like a tampon with lots of surface area and insert into the mother's vagina
3. Leave inserted for 1 hour and remove just prior to surgery and keep in a sterile container
4. Immediately after birth apply the swab to the baby's mouth and face, then to the rest of the body

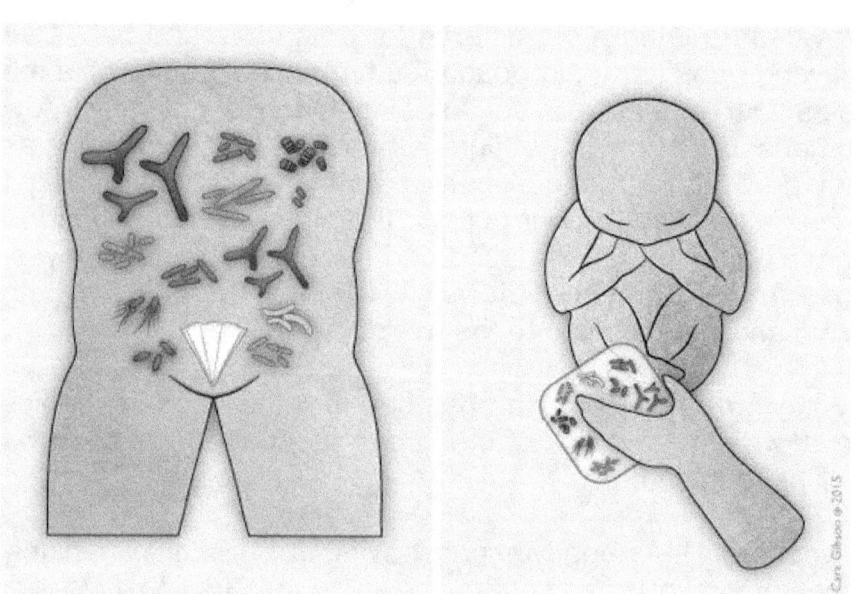

There is a great difference between the gut flora of a baby born vaginally compared to a baby born by c-section. As you read previously, during a vaginal birth the baby is colonized by your bacteria. A baby born by c-section is colonized by the bacteria in the hospital room; this leaves him with significantly less diverse bacteria than vaginally born babies. These differences could be behind the increased risk for specific diseases for babies born by c-section. (236)

Your baby's immune system needs your seeding. Research shows that after a mother's birth is interfered with, by use of pitocin, antibiotics, a c-section, or even formula feeding after birth, her baby may not be properly seeded. Without proper seeding, your baby's gut is left incomplete. This means your baby's immune system may never develop to its full potential. (237)

Did You Know?

The most beneficial gut bacteria are found in exclusively breastfed babies born vaginally, unmedicated and at home, after 37 weeks gestation. (236)

There are several ways in which you can help properly seed your baby:

- Have a vaginal birth in your own home environment.
- Avoid cervical exams.
- Avoid antibiotics during labor.
- If a c-section is needed, follow the seeding procedure (and exclusively breastfeed if possible!)

After birth, colonization of the baby continues through contact with the environment and breastfeeding. There are significant differences in the bacteria of breastfed babies compared to formula fed babies. Beneficial bacteria are directly transported to the baby's gut by breastmilk. (235)(239)(238)

After birth consider the following:

- Skin-to-skin immediately after birth and throughout infancy. The baby should be naked (or in a diaper) against your bare chest.
- Avoid bathing baby for at least 24 hours after birth, and avoid using soap of any kind on him until her is over 4-6 weeks old (or older). (240)
- Bring a blanket from home to wrap baby in at the hospital.
- Even with breastfeeding, consider taking a high quality probiotic.
- Avoid giving baby unnecessary antibiotics. If antibiotics are required, probiotics need to be considered. (241)

Chapter 32

VBAC
A Beautiful Journey

I applaud you. You are strong, informed, and looking to do things different with this birth.

I know that you are already holding a beautiful baby, but something about your previous surgical birth haunts you. Something says, "I want to do it different this time."

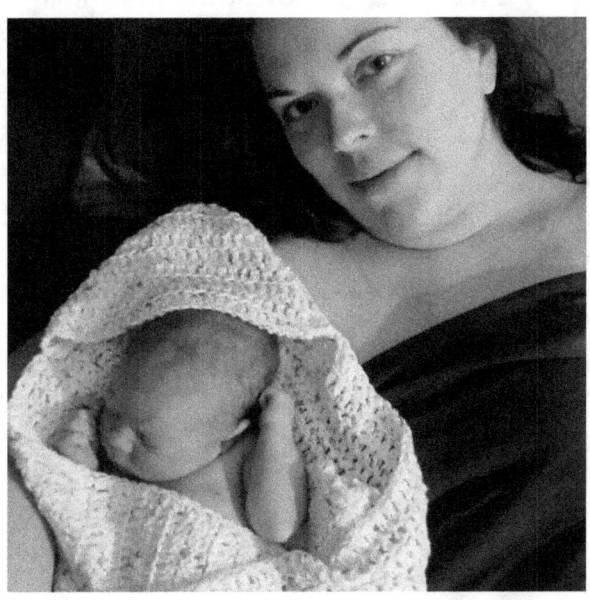

You can take charge of your pregnancy and birth. You CAN have a VBAC. Having worked with several couples striving for this goal, I have created a "To-Do List" for couples to complete on their beautiful journey to healing and accomplishing a vaginal birth.

Join the ICAN network: http://www.ican-online.org/

Reevaluate Your Previous Birth(s): Write it all down – everything about your birth that you remember. Try to include your emotions, physical experiences, and mental hurtles in as much detail as you can. Then you read it. Reread it over again – out loud. Then talk about the birth with your partner. From there, you can decide what exactly you would like to go differently this time. Were you induced, labor failed to progress, or baby was "too big?" This is time to learn the truth and figure out what you, your partner, and the birth team could have or should have done different.

Learn Your Fears and Emotions: If feelings of guilt, sadness, or fear arise while reliving your birth, that is ok. Talk to your current birth team about your feelings.

Find a VBAC Friendly Birth Team/Birthing Center: This is key to having a successful VBAC. Seek a midwife, if possible, who performs VBACs. A VBAC friendly birthing center is also ideal. If you feel comfortable, choose a homebirth. Eliminating the medical interventions is what will prevent the domino effect from beginning. If using an OB, make sure that he or she is understanding of your wants and is willing to work with you throughout the pregnancy to meet your goals.

Ask Questions/Get Answers: Do not be afraid to hunt for your perfect birth team. Talk openly and make sure that you are on the same page.

Take a Natural Childbirth Class: Yes, I will preach this every chance I can get. *Take a class.* A series of classes. Whether you want an unmedicated birth or a vaginal medicated birth, take the classes. You will build your confidence, lower your fears, and understand that you are capable.

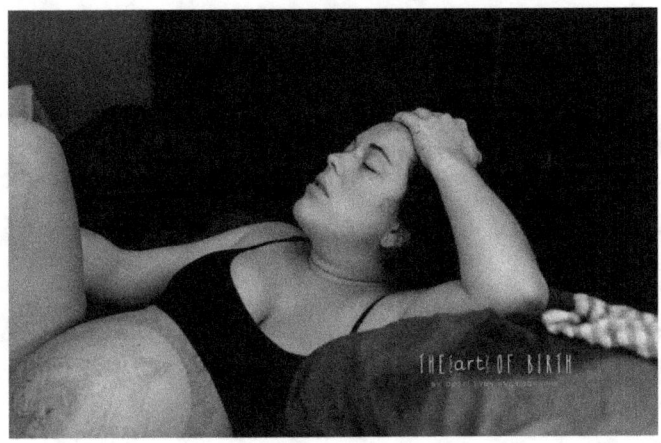

Read, Learn, and Know: Throughout your classes you will learn a lot about pregnancy, labor and birth, but don't stop there. Pick up a book or six. Read blogs and articles. Learn everything about every stage of labor and techniques to handle them, all of the best 2nd stage pushing positions, ideas for changing positions, techniques to speed up labor, and every way to practice relaxation. Understand what your body went through during your c-section and what will be different with a natural birth. Know your birth team and trust them. Learn about their ways and talk to them about yours. Allow yourself to soak it all in and enjoy the journey.

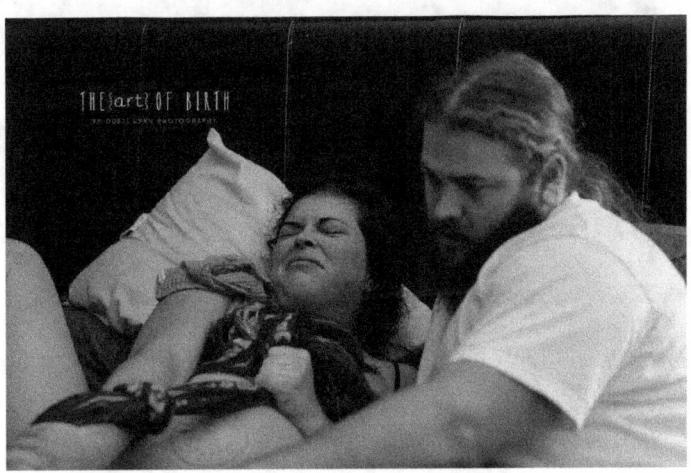

Visit a Chiropractor: Not only does getting adjusted relieve pregnancy ailments, but it helps baby align himself for birth, which will increase your successful VBAC chances! It's all about baby's position!

SpinningBabies.com: I have mentioned this site previously, but knowing your baby's position will help ensure your confidence in having a VBAC.

Hire a Doula: Having an experienced VBAC doula present is worth every single dime. She has the ability to help guide you through this beautiful journey! In fact, I highly, highly encourage you to hire a doula for any birth, but especially for VBAC

Practice Yoga: Inner peace is extremely important to ensure that your body is working with (not against) your baby.

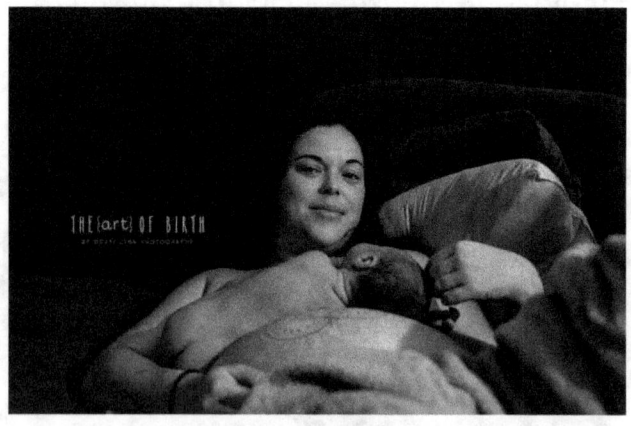

Did You Know?

C-sections are needed in the case of a transverse baby, complete placenta previa, and a few other circumstances that may become apparent during labor, such as cord prolapse.

A c-section is not needed as often as it is performed. Doctors may use reasons to surgically remove your baby, such as an estimated "big" baby, going past 40 weeks gestation, breech presentation, twins, water broken more than 24 hours. It is best to talk to your birth team about all or any other options.

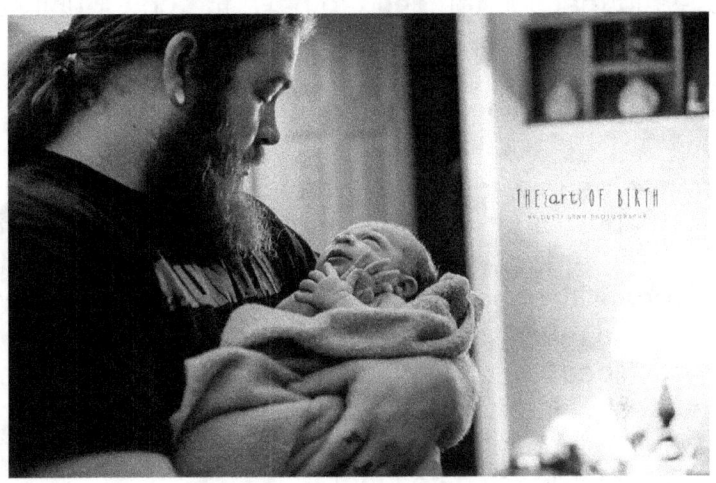

Chapter 33
Denying an Unnecessary Medical Induction

In our drive-thru society of getting everything we want when we want it, it comes as no surprise that so many women elect to be induced. I mean, how cool is it to pick your child's birthday? Not only that, but you get to end your pregnancy early!

I understand that it is tempting to have the opportunity to not go past your due date, avoid a certain date, share a birthday with a holiday, etc. but induction is not the smart choice; and research has proven it.

Doctors are people too. They have real lives. They have families, friends, and vacations that they want to be present for this year. Inducing their full-term patients allows them a higher probability of being in attendance. With everything that you have read thus far, I hope you understand just why this is not a good idea. Inducing your labor is the first step in a domino effect of interventions that can potentially lead to birth trauma, birth injuries, and unplanned c-section (In the moment known as "emergency c-sections").

Don't get me wrong. I do believe that medicine has its place, and medical interventions to birth are no exception; however, receiving an induction without medical necessity is asking for things to go wrong. There is a place and time when mothers truly need to be induced, and for those moments, I am so thankful for the medical capabilities. But, talk to any first time mother who voluntarily was induced, and you have more than a 50% chance of talking to a mom who was c-sectioned or experienced another form of birth trauma.

A recent study may help you decide against considering an induction. Australian researchers followed 28,000 women through spontaneous and induced labors. Results showed a 67% increase in c-section deliveries and a 64% increase in NICU care for women and their babies who chose an induction. (339)

When a normal labor is handled in a medicated fashion, it becomes a medical issue.

Some doctors conveniently have several common "medical" reasons to talk you into an induction:

- **Large Baby**: Too bad that the only way to truly diagnose macrosomia is after birth. Ultrasounds may be off by up to 2lbs, and the later in pregnancy that the ultrasound is performed, the less accurate the measurements are. Too often we hear about women electively having labor induced because the baby is too big, but in reality the baby is completely average. It is very, VERY rare that your body will grow a baby bigger than you can vaginally deliver.

- **Low Fluid Levels**: Fluid levels are of course important, but what doctors fail to mention is that your *amniotic fluid levels are directly related to your water intake.* If an ultrasound is showing lower than average fluid amounts, try to significantly increase your water intake and have another ultrasound preformed before agreeing to an induction.

- **A Multiple Pregnancy**: Yes, a birth of twins or triplets in our society is viewed as a higher risk than a singleton pregnancy. But you can still have a vaginal birth - on the day that your babies choose to be born. Multiple babies need as long as possible in the womb to grow. Labor will start when it is supposed to.

- **Previous C-Section**: If your doctor will not even let you go into labor on your own because you have had a previous c-section, many other doctors and midwives are open to VBAC's. You are capable of attempting and having a VBAC. The success of your VBAC will have a much higher probability if you allow your baby to truly be ready to be born.

- **Maternal Age:** Your age does not determine your baby's birthdate.

Agreeing to (electing) an induction can lead to many problems for your baby:

- A longer hospital stay after he is born or a visit to the NICU
- Remittance to the hospital
- Problems breathing
- Trouble regulating body temperature
- Feeding problems due to trouble sucking and swallowing
- Newborn jaundice
- A smaller and less developed brain

Even if your baby does well when born, he may have more long-term health problems such as:

- Attention Deficit Hyperactivity Disorder (ADHD)
- Increased risk of Autism (242)
- As an adult, he is more likely to have diabetes, high blood pressure or heart disease

The World Health Organization has declared 39 weeks full-term (instead of the previous 37 week label), but there is still so much happening at this point in pregnancy! To electively induce now takes precious days of growth away from your baby. During week 39 and afterward several important things are taking place: (243)

- Advanced muscle development is taking place: aiding with the suck and swallow motion of nursing

- Body temperature control is being moderated

- Further brain development is taking place

- Higher body fat is accumulating

- Advanced body system development and maturation is occurring: lung development, digestive system, nervous system, etc.

A due date is not written in stone. Electing induction at 39 weeks could place you at risk for delivering a baby that is not truly at 39 weeks gestation. Remember that your due date can be off by up to two weeks.

Did You Know?

When you wait for labor to begin naturally, you are lowering your chances of all of the following: (244)

- post-partum hemorrhage
- unplanned c-section
- jaundice
- respiratory problems
- seizures
- brain hemorrhage
- hearing issues
- medical interventions
- infection

Chapter 34

Naturally Inducing Labor

I have *SO MANY* clients approach 39-40 weeks begging me for ways to help get their baby out sooner than later. I sympathize and try to gently remind them that the end is near, pregnancy is not forever. There are those, though, who are staring at a medical induction at a certain date, or those about to risk out of their choice birth place due to going past a certain date on the calendar. To those clients, I start guiding them into all the ways to naturally bring baby earthside, including with my chiropractic help.

The biggest problem is that a baby WILL NOT COME if he is not ready. Induction will lead to c-section if your baby is not ready to be born. So please try to hold out and wait on baby.

* If you are in a position of 40+ weeks, and you are begging for ways to help get labor started before a doctor does, then read on.

The following are all natural ways to coax baby out of the womb, *if they are ready.*

Sex: Sex is a commonly suggested method of natural induction due to the semen containing prostaglandins, which help to ripen the cervix. Please note, that sex is safe throughout the entire pregnancy and is not linked to premature rupture of membranes or early labor; however, if your water has broken, do not have sex.

Chiropractic Care: Not only can your chiropractor ease symptoms during pregnancy, there is research that shows she can help with your labor too. Research found that women who receive chiropractic care during pregnancy have about 6 fewer hours of labor than women who do not receive this care. As you have read, your chiropractor can not only ease your pain, helps with inutero-constraint to help align the pelvis for baby to be in optimal position. (245) (246)

Nipple Stimulation: Stimulating the nipples (including your areola, as a baby would when sucking) triggers the production of natural oxytocin. Oxytocin contracts the uterus. You can stimulate by hand, orally, or with a pump, but only stimulate one nipple at a time. You can massage the first nipple for 5 minutes (when there are no contractions), then wait to see what happens (around 15 mins or so) before doing more. It's a good idea to take your mind off things by getting on with your usual duties than sitting and waiting for something to happen – so try and keep busy! Once labor is well established again, stop the stimulation.

Acupuncture: Acupuncture has been used for thousands of years to induce women who are 'overdue' in their pregnancy. Through continual research, it's been found that acupuncture generally works within 6-48 hours of having your treatment. (247)

Acupressure/Trigger Points: You can find a wonderful reference of acupressure for pregnancy and birth here: http://acupuncture.rhizome.net.nz/download-booklet/

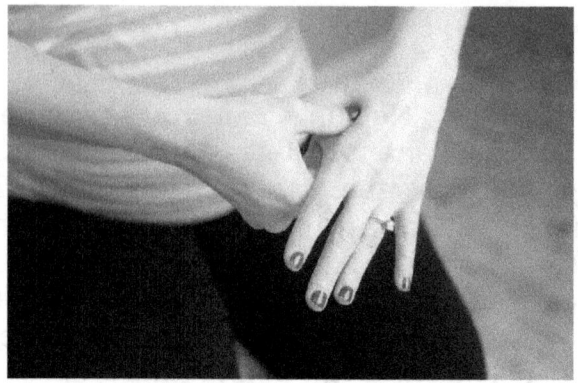

- To try inducing your labor, apply pressure between the thumb and index finger. This pressure point can be rubbed for several seconds or you can press it firmly for a minute.

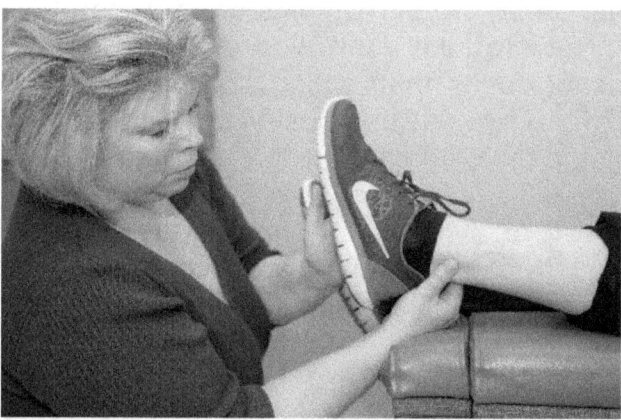

- Next, you will apply pressure to two different pressure points. The first point is located on the outside of the ankle. The other ankle pressure point is inside the leg, above the ankle. Make sure you find the correct placement of the points.

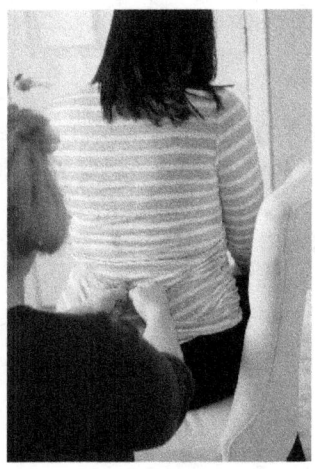

- The last point is located on the back, just above the butt on the lower back.

Homeopathy: *Pulsatilla* and *Caulophyllum* are two commonly used homeopathic remedies used to stimulate labor, but you should talk with your midwife about dosage.

Evening Primrose Oil: EPO may not induce labor, but it can prime and soften your cervix. You may take the oil orally or insert it vaginally for the best results. Again, talk with your midwife about dosage.

Red Raspberry Leaf Tea: RRLT can trigger contractions that may be able to start labor if your baby is ready. It is used more to tone the uterus and keep you hydrated.

Cinnamon stick tea - Take cinnamon sticks and boil them into a tea and drink. It actually tastes good so even if it doesn't bring on labor it may help you to relax!

Clary Sage Oil: Most midwives and doulas carry this essential oil with them for labors. It is known to promote relaxation and pain relief during labor. You can mix CSO with a carrier oil (like Coconut Oil) and rub on your pressure points before performing acupressure for best labor-inducing results.

Pineapple: Most tropical fruits such as pineapples, papaya, kiwi, and mango contain proteolytic enzymes. These enzymes break down protein and are thought to have medicinal properties. Pineapples have been used as to induce labor throughout the world for centuries. It is believed that bromelain, a type of proteolytic enzyme found in pineapples, may help to soften the cervix. Since pineapple may cause diarrhea, it is possible that it stimulates contractions as well.

Exercise: Walking on an uneven surface such as a curb or *lunging* up the stairs can help drop baby into a lower and more engaged position for labor to begin. *Squatting* reduces the birth canal by 10% and helps to get baby into the lowest position for birth.
Walking in general applies the pressure of your baby's head against your cervix and stimulates the release of oxytocin, which may bring on labor.

Castor Oil: Rubbing two tablespoons of castor oil on the belly (around the uterus) can possibly cause contractions, leading to labor.

Dates: Eating 6 dates per day for the last 4 weeks of labor have shown to have helped with shorter labor times and less Pitocin.(248)

Enemas or other bowel preparations (castor oil): I do not recommend this method, as it causes the bowels to contract, with hours of diarrhea resulting. The diarrhea causes dehydration, which can cause the uterus to contract – leading to labor. Please talk to your midwife or doctor before experimenting with drinking castor oil.

"There is power that comes to women when they give birth. They don't ask for it, it simply invades them. Accumulates like clouds on the horizon and passes through, carrying the child with it."
-Sheryl Feldman

Chapter 35
Labor Extremes: Precipitous and Prodromal

One of the most common misconceptions about labor is how long it lasts. It seems that the expected length is when it follows the not-so-normal bell curve that most assume labor to be defined by. They also expect to be dilating a centimeter an hour, and pushing immediately at 10 centimeters.

I'm sorry to tell you that this is far from true for so many birthing women. There are two reasons that doctors will tell you to expect labor to be around 12 hours. The first reason being the "dilate a centimeter an hour" thing and another 2 hours for pushing. (First time moms push over 2 hours on average, but that statistic includes medicated mothers). The second reason is that studies show an average birth lasts 12-14 hours in length. But you understand what 'average' means in the mathematical world - you add all the birth hours up and divide by the amount of mothers in the study(ies). So if the average is 12-14 hours, that means half of women will exceed that number and half will labor for far fewer hours.

In our society, women who do not follow the "normal" pattern are labeled as having 'complicated labors.' In all reality, there is no true 'normal' for birth, but instead, a normal for each mother and each baby's birth.

I want to talk about the two 'extremes' when it comes to labor length: Precipitous Labor and Prodromal Labor.

A labor is considered precipitous when it lasts three hours or less.

According to the CDC, just over 2% of births are truly precipitous deliveries. Although the data is only from women who reported their birth experiences. I assume it is safe to say the number is much higher than what is reported, as I don't think many women report their labor times. I would like to note that many women under chiropractic care tend to birth quickly because their babies are in optimal birth position.

There are no known causes to an extremely fast labor, but possible reasons you may birth quickly include: (249)(250)

- Family history of fast labor
- An extremely strong uterus
- A well-aligned pelvis and birth canal
- A baby positioned perfectly
- A smaller baby and a premature labor

Precipitous labor can come on like a freight train. Contractions are irregular, unpredictable, extremely intense, and never-ending. Handling these without fear is quite an accomplishment. If you are suddenly experiencing contractions one on top of another with little to no rest between them, your body is already transitioning and you need to prepare for the second stage: pushing. Pushing is not controlled. Your body will react without you helping it. The best thing to do is give in and gently aid your body and deliver your baby without panicking.

There are several challenges that come with having a precipitous birth. You may experience everything from self-doubt due to the intensity of the contractions to accepting an unprepared birth environment. A precipitous birth may occur on your bedroom floor with you digesting your emotions and processing the cycle of fear, but remember to breathe through it and stay as relaxed as possible. Work with your body, do not fight against it. Working with your body can help prevent tearing while pushing.

If you do experience a precipitous birth, please call your birth team the moment you think that your labor is happening faster than you expected. Never panic, birth is natural and you can do this. You and your partner should take a 'hands-off' approach to this birth; never pull on the baby, the cord or the placenta. Do not cut the cord; let nature work and bring your baby directly skin-to-skin.

On the opposite side of the spectrum, you may experience a labor long enough to make you doubt that it is even labor. This is known as prodromal labor, and there is nothing false about it.

Birth workers are quick to tell you that you are experiencing false labor, and often, it is discouraging. But the truth is that you are in labor. Your body is working hard to bring your baby into your arms. The best thing you can do is listen and work with it.

Many mothers who experience prodromal labor describe their experience in a similar way, although yours may not fall into this pattern. Steady, strong contractions begin each evening at the same time and last through the night but do not become stronger or closer together. It is exhausting and continual, happening every night for a week or more.

Intead of dismissing this stage of labor, birth workers have labeled it the 'latent phase.' While it can be long, tiring, confusing, and discouraging, know this: A latent phase typically leads to a shortened active labor. Your body does so much work preparing, that once your labor does intensify, it is ready to birth. Dilation, effacement and station position of the baby has already been progressing.

There is not one specific reason that you may experience prodromal labor, but instead many possibilities. You may have emotional or physical needs that must be worked out before labor will intensify. Emotionally, your body may be holding on to feelings, blocking its ability to focus on the task at hand. Physically, there is so much happening with your body and your baby:

- Baby is positioning for birth
- Baby lungs are being massaged with contractions
- Baby's nervous system is being activated
- Breastmilk is forming immunities
- Birth canal is aligning with pelvis

These things sometimes take much longer in some births.

Prodromal labor begins with contractions stronger than your typical Braxton Hicks, but they fail to get stronger. There may be true consistency and a regular pattern to your contractions, which is why so many women head to their place of birth; however, these contractions may not be regular at all. Don't you wish labor could be easier to understand? The latent phase may last a week or two with contractions coming for hours at a time and then ending. You may feel the need to limit your activities during your contractions, relaxing and working with your body to bring baby earthside. A warm bath may help you relax.

Seeing your chiropractor during your latent phase can be highly helpful in speeding things up. Many birth professionals feel that prodromal labor is the result of poor baby positioning. Sometimes a baby is positioned "sunny side-up" but wants to move into a more optimal position. Your body may begin to labor, using contractions to aid the baby in turning. This is a lot of work, so the body takes a break after a few hours and continues again later.

If positioning issues are truly the cause of your prodromal labor, you need to work with your body in every way possible. Chiropractic adjustments will help align everything and trigger active labor to begin. You can also try many exercises and positions to persuade your baby to move. Again, I recommend visiting www.spinningbabies.com, as it contains exercises and tips for every pregnancy and labor situation.

I also feel like having a doula on your side can really help you in these instances. You can look for the right doula for you at www.doulamatch.com or ask for recommendation as well.

As you can imagine, a prodromal labor can be challenging. I am not saying that it is more or less challenging than a precipitous birth, as they are both difficult to experience and digest afterward. I am saying though, that a prodromal labor has a higher chance of turning into a medical birth. It is completely possible to have a positive and natural birth experience with prodromal labor; the key is to rest as often as possible, trust in your body, and not let anyone take over, but instead have a supportive birth team who will work with you – not against you.

Prodromal labor is not a sign that your body doesn't work, but just the opposite. Your body is actively working -hard- to give you the healthiest natural birth possible.

Did You Know?

Psychological barriers, fears, and other emotions – even subconscious ones – may be holding your labor back. Utilize your birth partner to talk your way into the right mentality to give birth. Sleep, rest, breathe, bathe, and work on giving in to your labor.

Chapter 36
First Stage of Labor

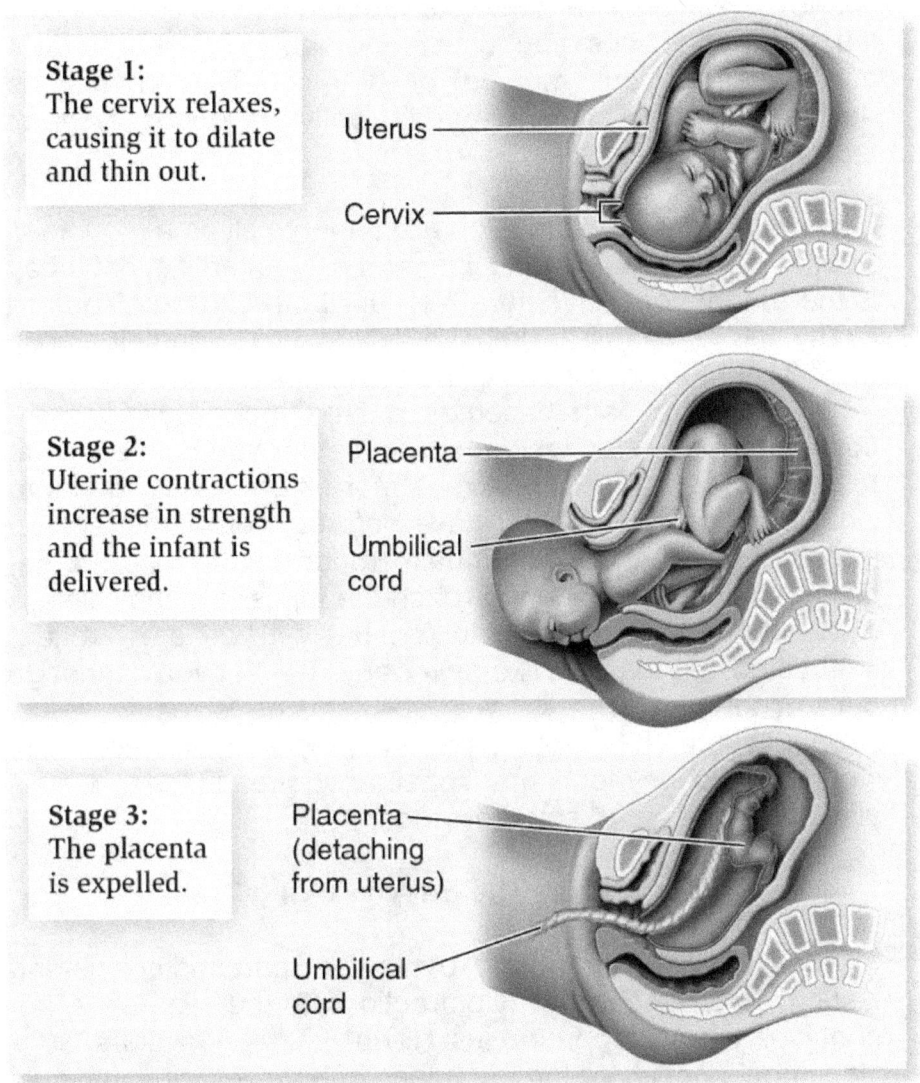

Stage 1:
The cervix relaxes, causing it to dilate and thin out.

Uterus

Cervix

Stage 2:
Uterine contractions increase in strength and the infant is delivered.

Placenta

Umbilical cord

Stage 3:
The placenta is expelled.

Placenta (detaching from uterus)

Umbilical cord

http://www.deluxechildbirth.com/getting-acquainted-with-the-3-stages-of-labour/

Labor is made up of three stages: the labor itself, pushing, and the birth of the placenta. Of course, each stage is then specific to each woman and her birth situation. The time you spend in each stage is completely dependent on your specific labor, the positions you choose to labor in, your baby's position, and your method of birthing. This chapter is dedicated to the first stage, and typically the longest stage of labor.

If you will, please imagine you are about to climb a mountain. Your support partner is with you, and as you realize that today is the day of your adventure, you are both excited. You are chatty and ready to go, almost overly exerting yourself across the ease of the flat ground. The elevation begins to increase slowly and the path becomes a little rocky, taking more concentration to stay on course. Together you both continue to climb. The trail only becomes more steep, causing you to work harder than you ever have before. You hit a place on the mountain that seems virtually impossible to hike. Forget hiking, the only way you will reach the top is to climb. This is what you have been training for, but yet you are terrified, exhausted, feeling pain like never before – but you cannot go back. Your partner is still with you, and he is ready. He is keeping you both hydrated, safe, and focused. Together you work to climb the mountain. Together you reach the top. This visual depicts the 1st stage of labor.

Early Labor: The Easy Walking Trail.

Your contractions are about 10 minutes apart and consistent, lasting 45-60 seconds. (Contractions further apart are not considered early labor, but just "Birth Prep contractions.")
You should not leave for your place of birth yet, as you would risk stalling your labor.

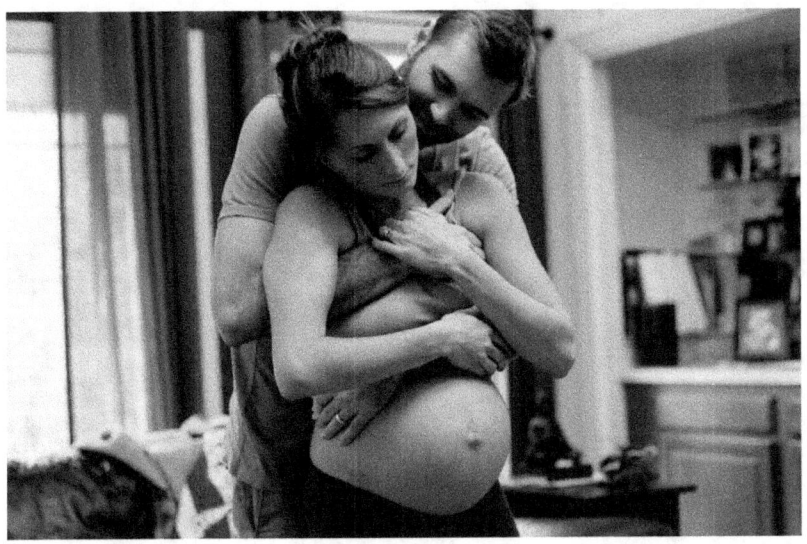

You should continue going about your daily routine and let the contractions come and go. You can call your partner home, but you can leave everyone else out of it for now. I wouldn't really call it labor until contractions are 10 minutes apart and consistent for at least 1-2 hours (or progressing faster). You may be anxiously cleaning, repacking your bag, prepping things for a homebirth, or just baking cookies, but remember to give in to each contraction and let it do its job. Some women can still talk and move through the contraction waves at this point, while others may be silent. Make sure to eat something during this stage; you will need energy throughout your mountain ahead.

During early labor, you may lose your mucus plug or find blood in the toilet. This is known as the 'bloody show.' There is absolutely no cause for alarm unless the bleeding is heavy and continuing. Contractions will typically last 45-60 seconds in length and progressively become more intense throughout labor.

You may feel better to move between contractions during this stage. The body is going through many changes, including:

- The brain observing what antibodies are needed in your breastmilk to allow your baby the exact right nutrients needed for this environment
- Your baby's nervous system and lungs are being prepped with each contraction

- Your body is moving baby down into an ideal birthing position.

If you are feeling tired at all, nap or rest. You are going to need all of your energy. But if you are well rested and ready to have your baby, walk and squat. Walking opens the inlet of the pelvis and squatting shortens the birth canal.

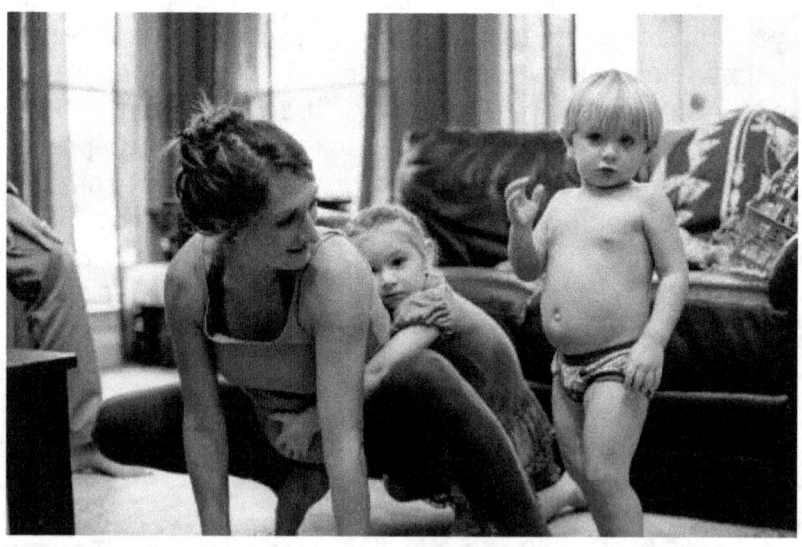

Try to keep your emotions in balance. Adrenaline can stop labor at this point, so being overly excited may delay your birth. Emotions are a huge part of this experience. Do not become discouraged if contractions taper off; your body will start working toward labor again within the next few days (or sooner). Breathe, you will meet your baby soon.

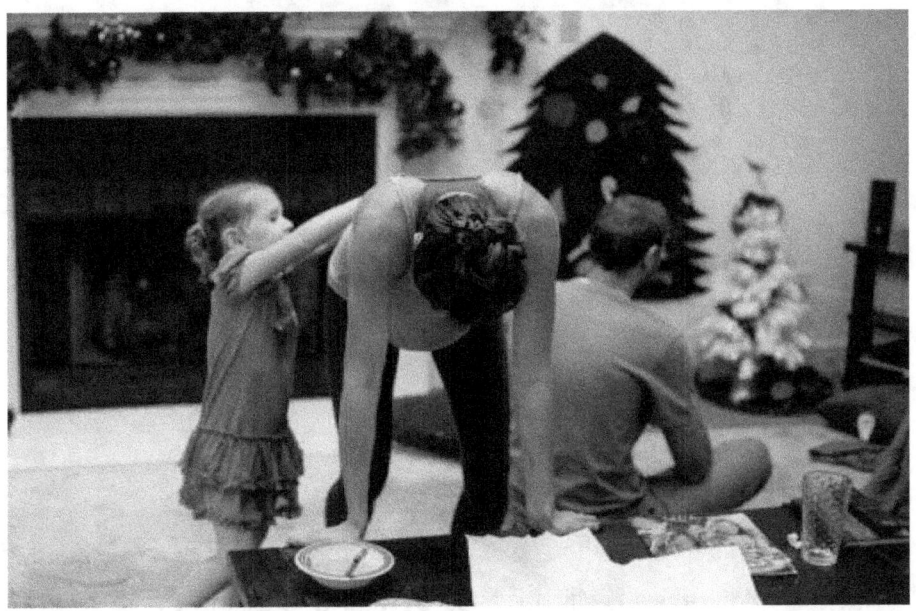

Active Labor: There's no turning back.
Your contractions are about 5 minutes apart, lasting around 60 seconds and intensifying.

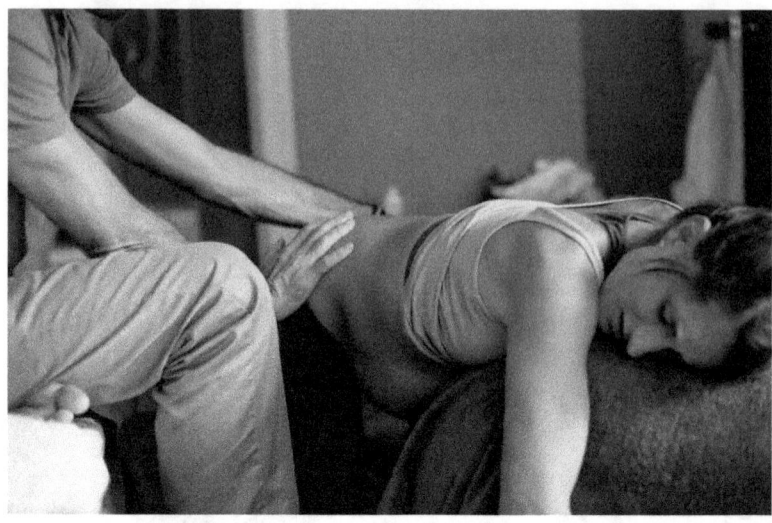

You can call your birth team once active labor has been consistent for an hour or so. No need to rush anywhere yet, but let them know you are progressing.

"This is it," becomes your thought process. You know you are in labor and that your baby will be here (relatively) soon. You will be working harder through the contractions at this point and may find one or two positions that work really well to handle the waves of tightness. Walking is still important, and you should be able to move and interact with others normally in between the contractions. Your support partner should continue making you eat and drink, and make sure your urinate often, as your full bladder can prolong labor. You will feel increasing pressure and fullness in your pelvis as active labor progresses, your back may ache, and a general crampy feeling may occur. I recommend sitting on a yoga/birth ball and rocking. The pelvis will be stretching and pulling, so rocking will help. Stay distracted in between contractions, there may be quite a journey ahead of you.

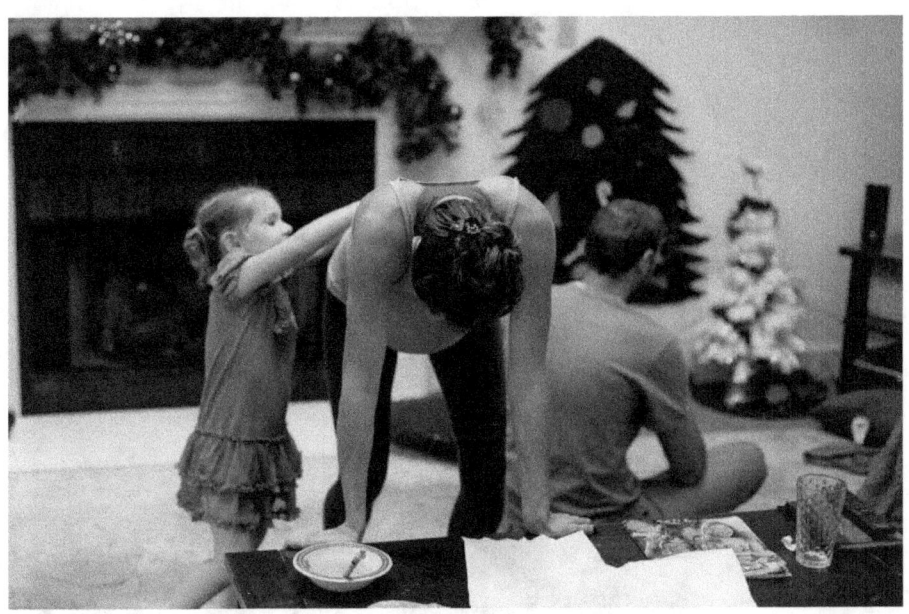

Contractions will become more intense and come closer together. As you enter late first stage of labor, you will become very serious and start losing your modesty. Your movements will become slower and more deliberate. A lot of women feel the need to lie down and build a "nest" – a quiet, cool, dark, comfortable place and ride out the intensity of the contractions. Close your eyes and mimic sleep. Breathe and use your relaxation techniques (that you have been practicing throughout your pregnancy). Your partner should be supporting you in any way possible: back rub, music, etc.

This is the time to leave for your place of birth.

If your water has not broken yet, now is about when it may. On average, it breaks near 8cm dilated or during the transition phase. Your water does not have to break, a baby born 'in the caul' is considered lucky.

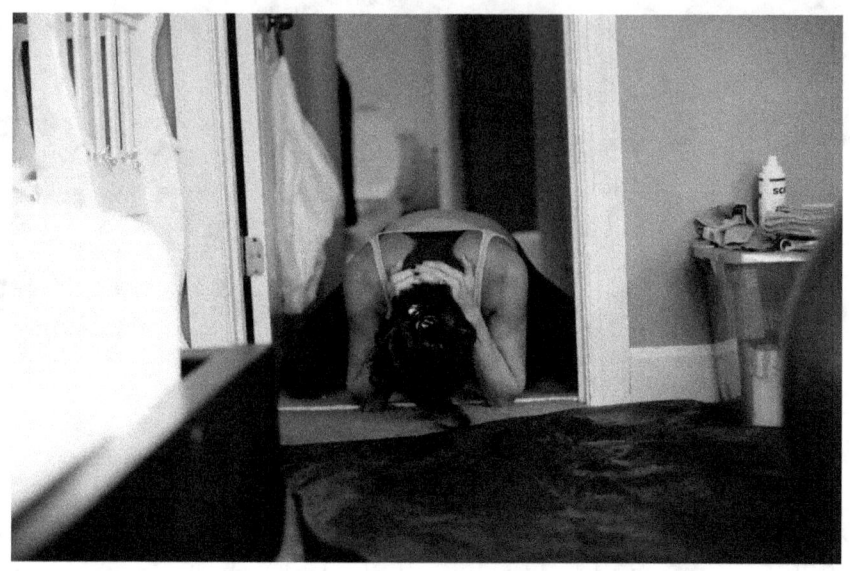

Transition: The uphill climb.

Your contractions are now irregular with double peaks, so intense, and all encompassing.

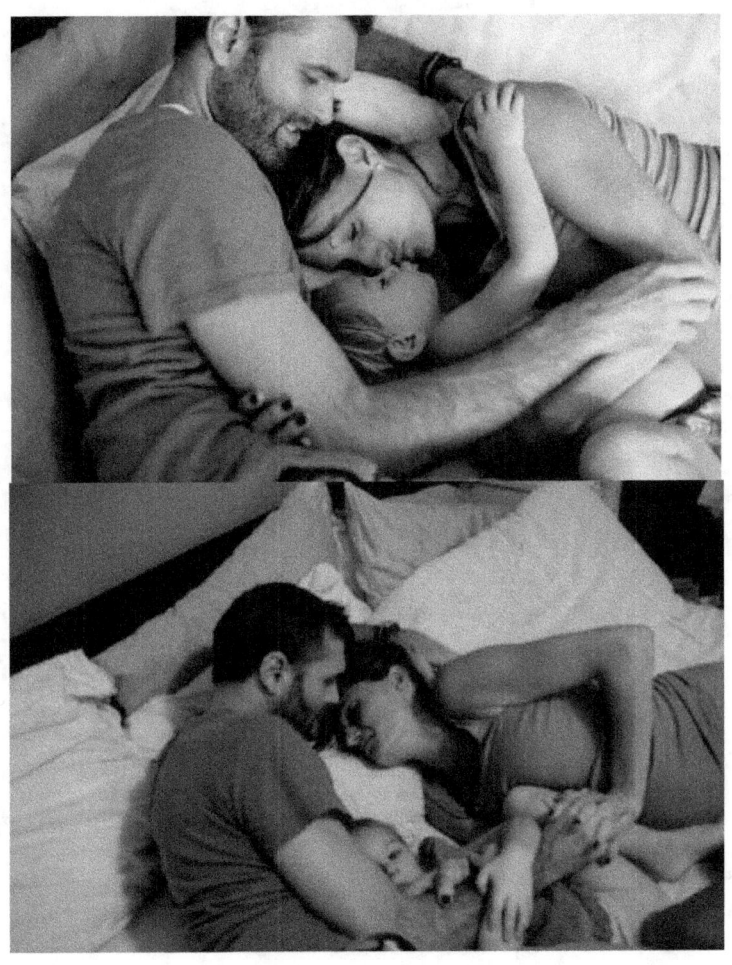

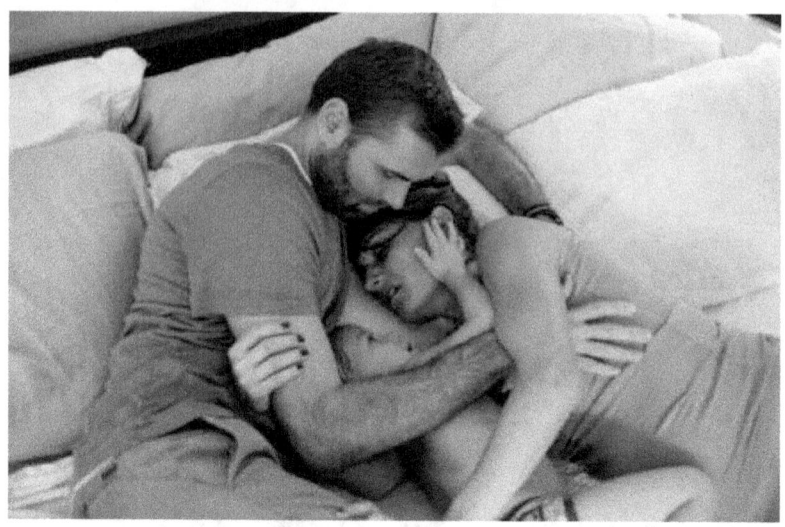

Inevitably, you will doubt your capability. This is how your partner will know you are transitioning. Transition is the point of labor when contractions become so intense that unprepared women beg for medical interventions. But if you are prepared and know what to expect, and know that transition is typically the shortest part of labor, you will give in to the contractions and allow your body to bring your baby into pushing position.

Transition can be viewed as the most raw and animalistic part of birth. You may feel like you are not present in your body even. There is no turning back though, and fighting the contractions will do nothing but intensify the moment. Have your partner repeat a mantra that you have chosen, such as, "Give in to your body and breathe our baby out."

Did You Know?

Knowing how far dilated and effaced you are will do nothing but terrify or aggravate you. You can go from 1 to 6cm in 5 minutes and in one contraction or it can take you three days to dilate 5cm. It means absolutely nothing. As long as you are contracting, your labor is progressing. Your body will naturally begin pushing once you are dilated enough to birth your baby. Every cervical check increases the risk of infection to you and your baby.

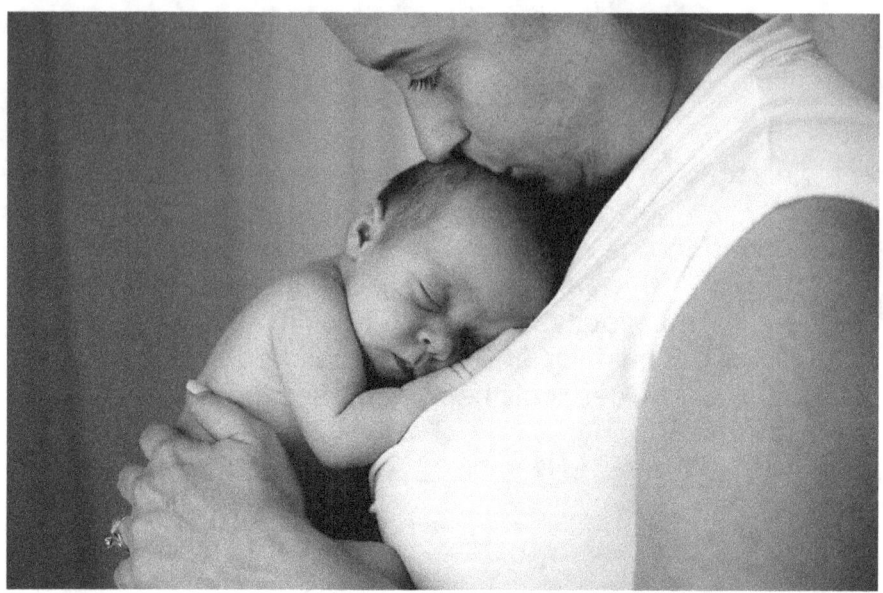

"Birth is not only about making babies. Birth is about making mothers – strong, competent, capable mothers who trust themselves and known their inner strength." -Barbara Katz Rothman

Chapter 37
Labor: 2nd and 3rd stages

There is a huge change in your labor once transition is complete. As the name describes, it transitions you to the next phase: pushing.

2nd Stage of Labor: Meeting your baby.

Your contractions will spread out and you will feel pressure to push. The pain and intensity of the 1st stage is now gone. You can breathe and relax again.

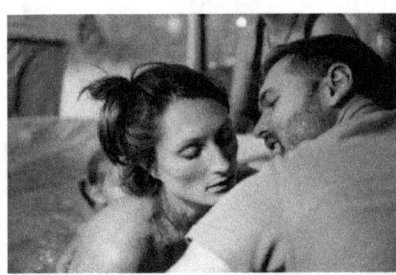
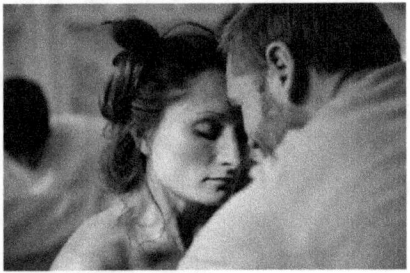
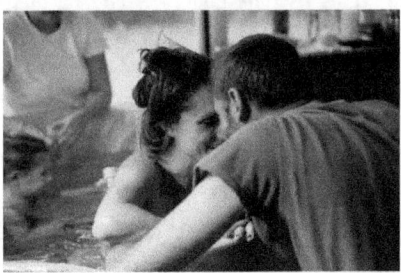

The easiest way to give in to pushing is to wait until your body pushes *ON ITS OWN* before you help baby out. It doesn't matter if the doctor says, "It's time to push." Pushing before your body is pushing is a huge waste of time. This is why most women push for hours.

After transition, the body will naturally give you a break. The contractions spread back out and become less intense. The waves become less of a painful tightening and more of a downward pressure. You'll feel pressure on your rectum and think pushing will help, but I beg you wait. Relax, sleep, and celebrate how far you have come.

There are several positions to birth in, and finding the right one for you and your baby is what is important. You do not want to give birth flat on your back. The amount of wasted energy spent there is exhausting. While pushing, your tail bone and pelvic bones shift, allowing baby to pass. If you are lying flat on your back, this process is nearly impossible and takes time and energy that should not be wasted.

You can give birth while on your side, on your hands and knees, squatting, standing, leaning, or in any position that is proving to be aiding your baby's birth. You may also change positions in between contractions

You will know when your body pushes. You may feel a burning sensation; this is the baby's head passing through the cervix.

Did You Know?

You or your partner can 'catch' your baby. The umbilical cord is the perfect length for your baby to be placed directly on your chest, while the placenta is still inside of you.

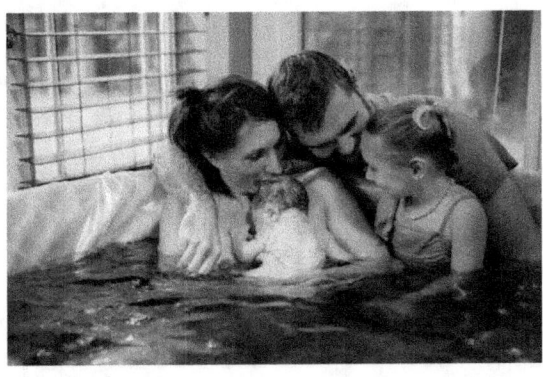

3rd Stage of Labor: Placenta Delivery

Many mothers don't remember delivering their placenta. Once you are holding your baby, everything else may seem to not exist. The cord does not need clamped or cut before the placenta is delivered, but it is important that your birth team makes sure the entire placenta has been birthed and not a piece was left attached to the uterine wall. If you feel feverish, your milk does not come in, or you start to feel ill within a few days after delivery, call your OB immediately.

Take a few minutes to really look at your placenta. This organ GREW A BABY inside of you. It is incredible!

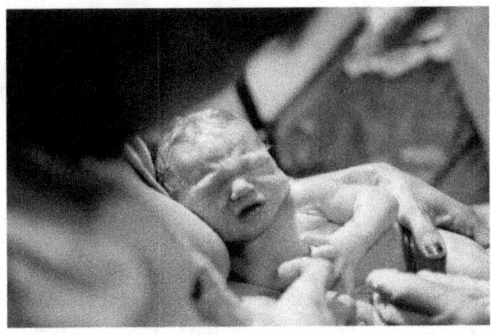

Chapter 38
The Placenta After Birth

There is no way that such an amazing organ is actually useless once the baby is brought earthside, but yet at most births it is thrown out as hazardous trash. There is so much goodness left though! The placenta's benefits continue even after your baby is born.

Your newborn should be placed on your chest skin-to-skin immediately after birth. This initializing breastfeeding and triggers contractions that aide in the delivery of the placenta. This is a time for bonding a und should be uninterrupted.

As the body initiates the contractions for the third stage of labor, the placenta deflates and detaches from the uterus wall. At the point of attachment, a clot forms to prevent bleeding.

The delivery of the placenta should not be rushed. You want the placenta to detach cleanly without leaving any of the little "branches" behind that connected it to your uterus. If they remain, they can prevent your uterus from being able to shut off blood supply to the placenta (that has already been expelled). The remaining 'branches' hold the same blood vessels open that were needed to keep the placenta and baby healthy in utero. This open blood supply then prevents the start of milk production and causes confusion within the mother's body – Are we still pregnant? When this occurs, it is called a retained placenta, and it can cause many problems, worse than your milk not coming in. If fever or flu like symptoms have begun within a week after birth, seek medical attention immediately.

Every placenta is different and unique to the mother and baby. Make sure that you inspect yours after birth!

Delayed cord clamping is important and being practiced more regularly now. After all of the amazing, healthy blood has finished passing from the placenta to your baby (You can actually watch your baby get pinker during this time!), the cord is cut and the placenta can be placed on ice to be taken home.

The most common practice in our society is to encapsulate the placenta. The act of encapsulating the placenta has been practiced across the world for centuries. Many cultures believe the nutrient-rich placenta will assist the mother in recovering from childbirth.

Placental encapsulation is the practice of ingesting the placenta. It can be steamed, dehydrated, or ground and placed into capsules.

A certified encapsulator thoroughly cleans any clots or blood from the placenta, and then, depending on the method chosen, the placenta may be steamed (with or without herbs), or it may go straight to being dehydrated. Once dehydrated, it is ground and put into capsules for you to take. It is taken as needed, typically within 2-3 days of birth, and then daily to rebalance your hormones. You can save capsules for when your period returns -or even for menopause.

Make sure you store your capsules in the refrigerator or freezer, but not near anything that could cause them to get wet.

Having your placenta encapsulated allows you to enjoy the following benefits: (251) (252) (253) (254)

- 14 trace minerals can be found within the encapsulated placenta. (255)
- General pain reduction (256)
- Decreased risk of post-partum depression
- Rebalanced hormone levels
- Increased release of oxytocin, which helps the uterus return to its normal size
- Increase in CRH, a stress-reducing hormone
- Rebalanced iron levels
- Increased milk production
- Increased energy
- Lessened postpartum cramping
- Lessened postpartum bleeding
- Normalized libido
- Increased bond with your baby
- Reduced stress levels
- Reduced swelling

Up to 80% of women experience the baby blues within the first week of birth. Women who consume their placenta report fewer emotional issues and a more enjoyable babymoon. (257)

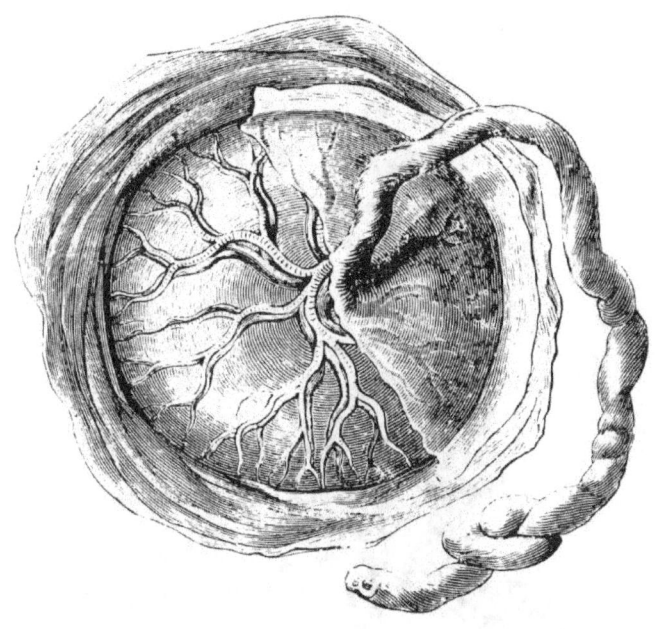

Did You Know?

There is more you can do with your placenta; you can also:

- Make a Placenta Print
- Placenta Tincture
- Placenta Smoothie
- Plant it
- Placenta Salve

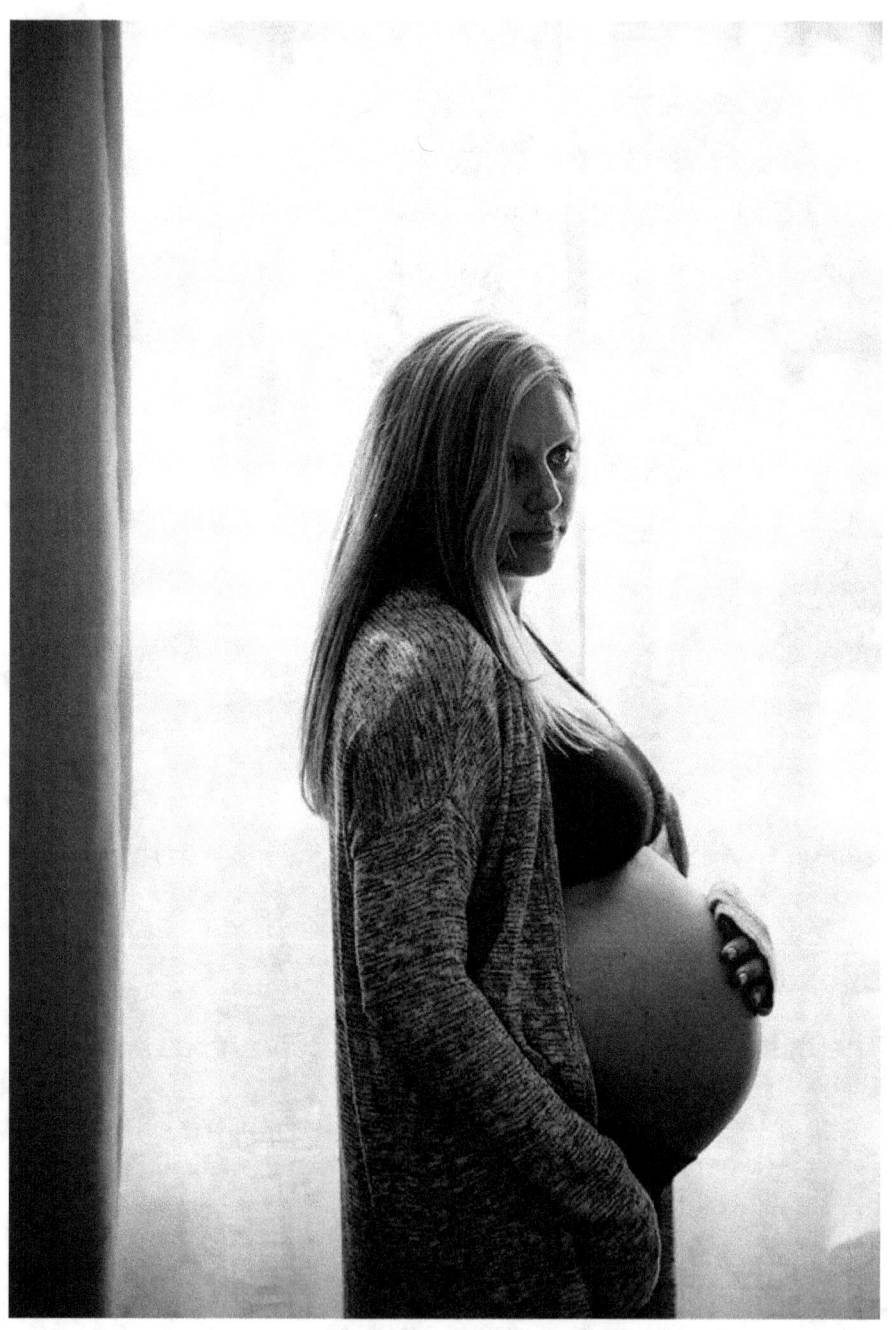

"If I don't know my options, I don't have any." - Diana Korte

Chapter 39
Domino Effect of Interventions

I hope you are understanding just how much of a conveyer belt society we are living in. While this theory benefits no one, it can do great harm to laboring women. It's as if pregnancy is a game of dominos instead of a natural supported aspect of life. The dominos are set up from the moment you conceive – the first appointment even. There are chances throughout your pregnancy that you are set up to lose this game, and if not while pregnant -then during labor. If the pieces cannot be stopped, the game ends in a traumatic birth experience.

Your birth may or may not be traumatic, or end in a c-section, but it has been found that one medical intervention tends to lead to another. Labor should not be intervened with – it is meant to be handled just as your body handles it.

There is a huge need for medicine – and doctors – when it comes to birthing. But the need lies with pregnancies that are not healthy or normal, those that are high risk. But for those of you with a healthy, low risk pregnancy, there is absolutely no need for medical intervention. Statistically speaking, a low risk pregnancy has a higher chance of ending differently than expected if even one intervention is allowed. Your place of birth and your birth team play a huge role in this also.(258) (259) (260)

One of the biggest problems is that most women do not know what an intervention is. They assume that interventions are the extremes – the epidural, the forceps, the c-section – and that they are only utilized when absolutely necessary. The truth is that the dominos begin to fall long before this, and that even the smallest interventions may lead to less "needed" end results.

Even being made to lay on your back while laboring is an intervention, as it interferes with your labor and goes against what the body naturally wants to do.

Once you realize how many interventions are available, you will then begin to prioritize just what you want, and what you are willing to let go of, to achieve your natural birth.

- Inducing labor in any form
- Having a cervical check
- Scraping the membranes
- Breaking the bag of water
- IV
- Pitocin
- Laughing Gas
- Epidural
- Catheterization
- Laying on your back (Squatting position is best)
- Feet restrained (held or in stirrups)
- Episiotomy
- Forceps assisted delivery
- Vacuum extraction
- Internal Fetal Monitoring
- Continuous external fetal monitoring
- Elective C-Section
- Repeat C-Section

These are just a few examples of medical interventions. (261)(262)

While some women are denying interventions, most are not; and
research shows that these 'routine interventions' can lead to unwanted and potentially harmful complications and outcomes. Once one medical procedure is preformed, a domino falls – into another – this leads to another, and another; the side effects of which create a condition that then requires more medical procedures.

Many who opt for the epidural will end their birth in the operating room or with an instrumental assisted delivery (forceps or vacuum). It will not happen to everyone, but an epidural increases cesearean section risk and vacuum or forceps extraction rates, especially in first time mothers. And of course these interventions can then lead to lifelong problems with you or your baby. (264)

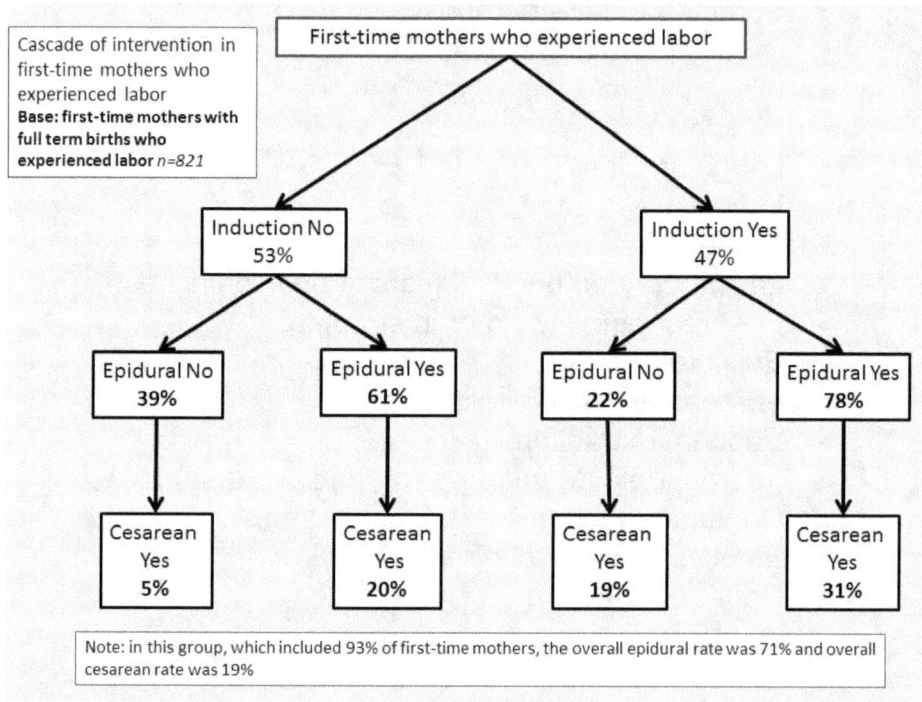

Cascade of intervention in first-time mothers who experienced labor
Base: first-time mothers with full term births who experienced labor *n=821*

First-time mothers who experienced labor

Induction No 53%

Induction Yes 47%

Epidural No 39%

Epidural Yes 61%

Epidural No 22%

Epidural Yes 78%

Cesarean Yes 5%

Cesarean Yes 20%

Cesarean Yes 19%

Cesarean Yes 31%

Note: in this group, which included 93% of first-time mothers, the overall epidural rate was 71% and overall cesarean rate was 19%

It is all about education. You need to know the domino effect before it happens so that you can plan your birth plan correctly. Knowing that any cervical exam can lead to infection, breaking the bag of water also puts you at risk for infection, and puts your labor on a clock, counting down to a c-section if baby does not arrive in a certain amount of hours. An epidural can lead to permanent back pain, dizziness, headaches, migraines, and leg pain, on top of the increased birth risk statistics. The more you educate yourself, the easier it is to make decisions in the moment. You will be able to prioritize and end the domino effect before it begins.

A c-section is typically what mothers want to avoid, but yet interventions can paint them into a corner quickly. In the past 40-50 years, our cesarean rate has skyrocketed! In 1965 the rate was less than 5%, today it is over 32%.

According to the World Health Organization, no country is should have a cesarean rate greater than 10%. Even the American College of Obstetricians and Gynecologists admits our statistics troubling. Our current statistics are higher than most other developed countries.

Even scarier than your birth resulting in a c-section, is your birth resulting in your death. It sounds like a horrible threat, however, the United Sates has an almost unbelievable rate of maternal mortality after birth. It has been found that a woman's risk of death during delivery is five times higher during cesarean than a natural delivery, an African American mother is 10 times more likely to die. According to the World Health Organization (and several United Nations agencies) we rank behind no less than 40 other nations in preventing maternal deaths. (264)

But why are our numbers rising and not falling? We live in a time when medical options should be our last resort – our saving grace. I believe that having unsupportive birth care during pregnancy and birth is playing a huge role in our statistics. Along with uneducated and unaware mothers, medical interventions laying claim to most, and our "one-size-fits-all" mentality, there is no reason for our rates to decrease.

It is time to change this.

Please understand just what is being risked when a c-section is performed, even when it is needed (265)These risks to you, the mother, include:

- Hemorrhage
- Hysterectomy
- Blood clots
- Delayed milk production
- Infection
- Bowel obstruction
- Severe and prolonged pain
- Scaring
- Re-hospitalization
- Postpartum depression
- Birth trauma
- Altered initial bond with your baby
- Future eptopic pregnancies
- Reduced fertility
- Future placental problems such as previa or abruption
- Stroke
- Ruptured uterus
- Death

Risks to your baby include:
- Preterm birth
- Low birth weight
- Breastfeeding struggles
- Breathing difficulties
- Asthma
- Abnormal or injury to the brain

While this all sounds scary and almost unavoidable, that is not the case. You can avoid medical interventions, and you can stop the dominoes from falling. I suggest having a supportive environment throughout pregnancy and birth. You can choose to be surrounded by people you trust. A midwife is your best option, but you can find aa doctor who supports VBACs, vaginal births, unmedicated births, and births with a hands-off approach. Hiring a doula can be your saving grace.

Make sure that you share your wants with your family and help educate them in your reasons so they feel connected and confident in supporting you.

I urge you to ask questions, weigh your risks and rewards with each decision, ask for options, buy yourself time to discuss, change positions and make the best choices for you.

Did You Know?

ACOG or American College of Obstetrician and Gynecologists recommend low-rick women that are progressing normally with no evenence of fetal compromise may not have to have a routive amniotomy, continuous fetal monitoring or IV fluids, can labor in ant position, and can drink water. (342)

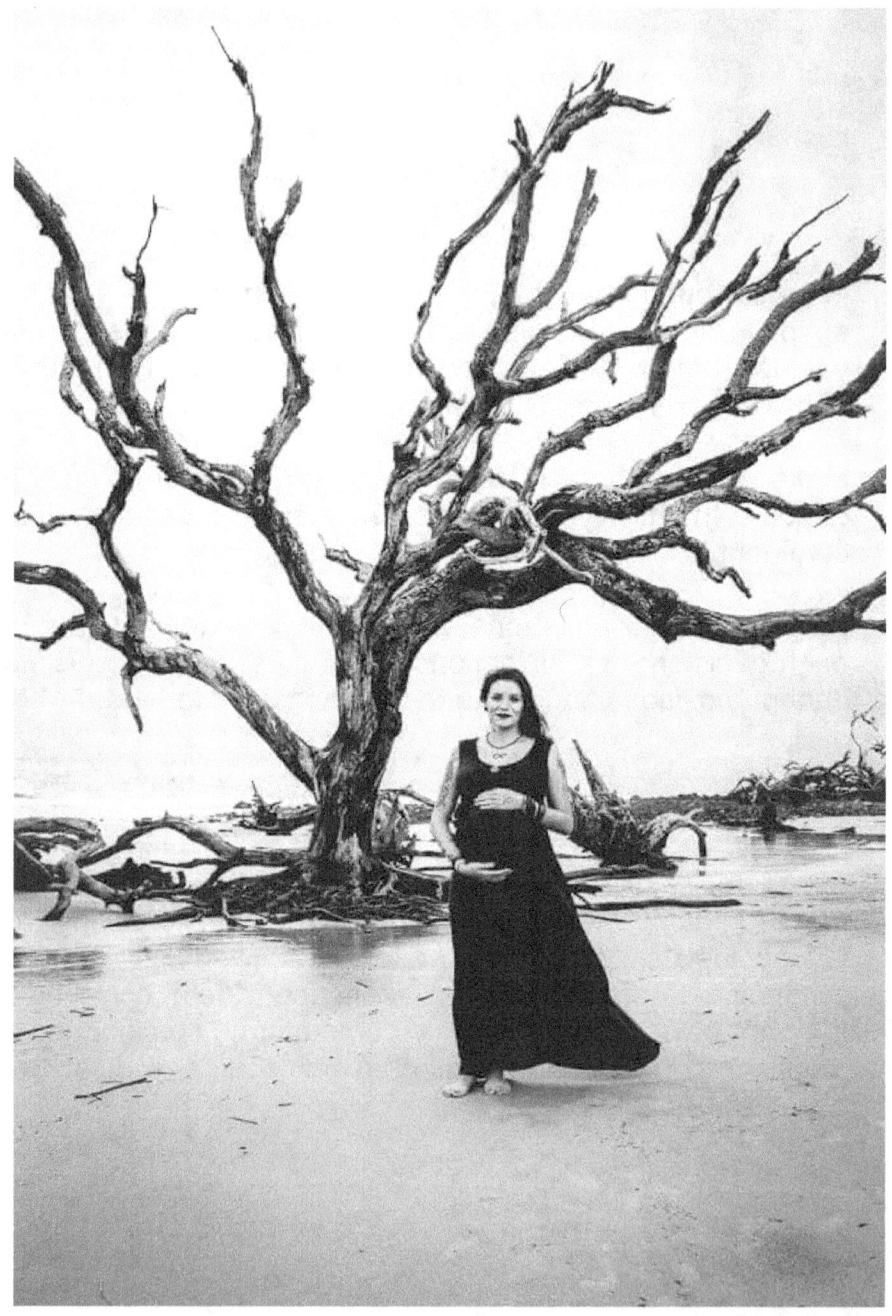

"We have a secret in our culture and it is not that birth is painful. It's that women are strong."
-Laura Stavoe

Chapter 40
Common Complications of Labor

It's funny. You rarely hear a home birth mother or midwife mention the word "complication" when it comes to labor. Doctors are meant to look for problems, not to support the norm. They tend to make problems arise, while many are trying to let moms naturally birth, that is not the case with all OBGYN. That is why it is imperative to research your birth team

While there are several causes for true complications, most of the time the complication terms thrown around in the delivery room are just that: words. The problem is that these words tend to then dictate the rest of the labor and possibly cause a real complication (remember the domino effect you just read about?).

To avoid any unnecessary stress or interventions, the best thing you can do is understand what constitutes a true complication. I have compiled a list of terms that are used and what the stand for; I'm also including options and natural ways to avoid interventions if any of these 'complications' should arise during your labor.

Overdue: Labor is not a predictable science. It is not supposed to be. A due date is an estimation and should be a "due month" with a four-week window (38-42 weeks). Your baby needs time to grow and develop and should not be taken any earlier than is needed.

Group B Strep: Taking the antibiotics are up to you. Be informed and make the right decision for your family.

PROM (Premature Rupture of Membranes): I will go into more detail soon, but this is when the water breaks before the onset of labor. Most birth locations will require you to birth within 24 hours of your water breaking. Remember that you do not need to notify anyone the moment your water breaks, or give a specific time. Waiting until contractions start and progress into active labor is the best thing to do.

AROM (Artificial Rupture of Membranes): This term may be used when trying to speed up your labor. It is when the doctor breaks your bag of water artificially. There is no need to break your water. While it may speed things up, perhaps your baby needed the extra time?

OP (Occiput Posterior): A baby who is "sunny-side up" – or looking up instead toward your back, is an OP baby. This position often causes very intense back labor but is not reason for any intervention. OP births are typically longer births because your baby needs more time to pass through the birth canal. Get into all 4 position and begin doing cat and cow yoga positions.

Breech: This refers to a baby who is feet or bottom down. Most cultures believe this to be a natural birth position, but in our society, you will find it hard to locate a doctor willing to deliver your baby vaginally while breech. Breech births require a hands-off delivery, as you should not pull on the baby at all. Wait for labor to start naturally and request an ultrasound during active labor before agreeing to a surgical birth.

Transverse Lie: This is when the baby has positioned himself horizontal, across the uterus instead of head down. While most transverse babies turn in labor, there is a chance the baby will not. This is cause for immediate intervention. Cesarean sections save mothers and babies in this situation!

 TVP (Transverse Vertex Presentation): This means that the baby's head is sideways. When in labor, baby should safely turn correctly, BUT an ultrasound is needed to ensure proper placement. A cesarean section will be needed if baby does not turn during active labor.

Precipitous Labor: Your birth team may recommend an immediate epidural to slow things down and get control of labor. But you have read that true fast labor will be too fast for interventions.

Prodromal Labor: As you have read, this is a long, slow, labor – but not need for intervention.

Reverse Dilation: This does not actually exist. Your cervix will not close during labor, it will only open. You may hear this term if:

- Two different people with different finger sizes do cervical checks
- The bag of waters was bulging against the cervix, but then breaks
- The baby changes position

Arrested Labor: A labor can stop for many reasons: fear, exhaustion, location change, and excitement, etc. True labor will start again, but it may take time for the body to adapt to the changes it experienced. Take the time to respect your labor.

NAP (Natural Alignment Plateau): Most doctors will use the NAP to labor a birth as one that is failing to progress. However it is a very normal part of labor; NAP is when labor contractions continue but dilation, effacement, and station stay the same. The body is still working, but a doctor sees little progress.

FTP (Failure to Progress): This basically means that you are not progressing as fast as your birth team would like you to. There are extreme situations when medical help is needed, but overall, the body is and will continue to progress on its own timeline. Do not rush things.

Extremely Painful Labor: Some doctors may refer to an

intense labor as extremely painful and recommend medical interventions to help the mother relax. Try changing positions. If there is a true reason for the pain (other than a normal labor), medical help could be needed.

CPD (Cephalopelvic Disproportion): This is a true reason for a c-section; however, it cannot be known until you are pushing. CPD is when the baby's head is larger than your body can birth. Changing positions to a squat or staggered squat (one leg on a chair) should help.

Multiple Births: The body is able to naturally birth twins or triplets (or more) just as it is able to birth a single baby. You do not need to schedule an induction or a c-section. Even you are backed into a corner and must have a surgical birth, you can fight for it to be done once labor begins naturally, this way you know your babies are ready to be born.

Prolapsed Cord: This is dangerous and terrifying. A prolapsed cord is when the umbilical cord exits the birth canal before the baby. It is cause for immediate medical intervention.

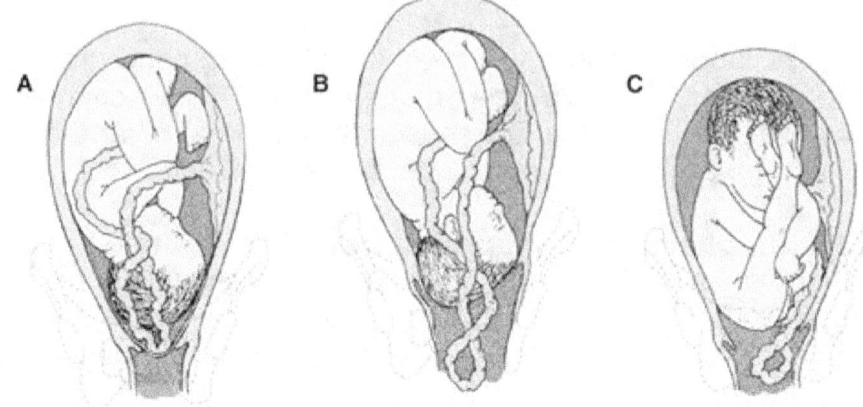

Lowdermilk, DL, and others. (2012). *Maternity and Women's Health Care, 10th Edition.* St. Louis: Mosby. Retrieved October 31, 2013, from Mosby's Skills

Placenta Previa: Another cause for medical intervention. The placenta cannot be birthed prior to your baby. A full previa is when the placenta is covering the cervix, which makes it impossible to birth your baby naturally. A c-section is needed.

Meconium Staining: Meconium is the first bowel movement from the baby. It may happen while still in the womb or during labor, but there is no need to panic. Current research disproves the outdated tradition of intervening with a birth due to meconium staining – poop in the amniotic fluid, especially if birth occurs between weeks 37-42. 15-40% of babies are born with meconium stained fluid. It has been proven that this meconium is not cause for hyproxia, and that most babies born in poor condition do not have meconium stained amniotic fluid (MSAF)– and most babies born with MSAF are healthy. (266)

An abnormal heart rate is a much better predictor to fetal

distress; and this along with meconium in the water may be truly be a sign of trouble. (267)

Meconium Aspiration Syndrome (MAS): MAS is an extremely rare complication. It is believed to occur when an *already hypoxic* baby gasps for air before he is actually born, but instead inhales meconium into his lungs. One research study suggested that most cases of MAS are not related to the aspiration of meconium, but instead to other extreme developments in utero, such as infection or chronic asphyxia. (268)

A healthy baby does not inhale amniotic fluid during labor.

Fetal Distress: I wish doctors (and all birth teams) would learn to not throw this term around so easily. If there is time to talk about options and discuss things, then it is not true distress.

When a true complication develops, it is cause for medical intervention. This is why our medical system exists. However, most things that women lose their birth plan to are avoidable.

Education is truly the key.

If a complication arises, your support partner should ask the birth team what the problem is and if you and the baby are currently okay. Take a minute to listen to the doctor and write things down. Once you have the information, talk together about your options. If you have a doula present, ask for her input. Keep your birth plan in mind and remember your priorities.

Did You Know?

Birth trauma or postpartum stress can arise from labor complications. Keeping a positive atmosphere during the birth is important, even if things are not exactly how you imagined them to be.

Chapter 41
P.R.O.M.

Premature Rupture of Membranes; the moment your water breaks but your labor has not yet begun, and you are at least 37 weeks pregnant. I am devoting a chapter to this 'complication' because it happens often. Your water may break before the onset of contractions. There is no need to panic, rush to your birth place, or start your stop watch.

Since the 1950's, doctors have placed women 'on the clock' when their water breaks.

This outdated policy still exists in hospitals and most birth centers across the country. It is purely liability purposes, which is sad because nothing actually happens at hour 25.

That's right. There are no sudden increased risk factors after 24 hours. (270) The clock does not dictate a medical emergency needing a c-section. There is absolutely nothing wrong with your body if it does not start labor immediately after your water has broken naturally. (Having your water broken by a doctor does not fall under this category. That is an intervention to your labor and should be avoided.)

The problem is that most women call or go into their birth place once their water breaks. Many doctors will begin to push for medical interventions (pitocin) if contractions are not present upon arrival. However, research shows that it is safer for you to allow the body to labor spontaneously. (269)

Studies show that 45% of women will naturally go into labor within 12 hours of their water breaking. (270) and over 75% of women will naturally go into labor within 24 hours (269) with over 85% of women going into labor naturally within 48 hours of their water breaking. Further research shows that women left to have labor begin on its own, have a significantly lower chance of receiving a c-section. (271)

We do not know how long a healthy labor can go before starting, as no documented births have been studied past 72 hours of water breaking.

Most women whose water breaks before labor begins do not have a specific risk factor linked to PROM. This means that it can happen to any mother without warning. However, there some factors that increase the chance of it happening to you. These factors include:

- Poor Nutrition
- Dehydration
- Smoking
- Infection (such as yeast infection)
- Prior cervical surgery
- Cervical exams - *Weekly vaginal exams starting at 37 weeks cause a three times higher chance of having PROM* (272)
- Having your membranes swept (273)
- Weakened amniotic sac (this may happen if there is too much fluid, or more than one baby putting pressure on the membranes) (274)
- If you were pregnant before and had a PROM or PPROM

There is, of course, the chance that your water breaks naturally before the start of labor, for no other reason than nature – it was meant to be. The membranes weaken towards the end of pregnancy, and the weakest part of the water bag can give out to Braxton Hicks contractions.

While there is no way to guarantee that you will not experience PROM, there are a few things you can do to help strengthen your bag of waters. Research links vitamin C to the strength of the amniotic sac. Increasing your vitamin C intake may help prevent PROM. There is also research linking high quality omega 3's and their ability to lessen inflammation to a decreased risk of PROM. (275) Avoiding all cervical exams is absolutely the best way you can try to prevent PROM. While it may be interesting to know if you are dilated, it truly means nothing in terms of your impending labor. Every vaginal check is a risk for infection, a link to causing another medical intervention, or a possible cause to PROM.

There are two problems that having your bag of waters broken may cause, but both are increased if labor is induced. The first problem is a drop in fetal heartrate. Babies whose water has broken are more likely to respond to contractions with a dipping heart rate, but as long as the heartrate recovers after each contraction, baby is okay. This is often the moment that a mother will be wheeled back for a c-section over "fetal distress." But, again, as long as the heartrate recovers between contractions, everything is ok.

The second problem linked to PROM is developing an infection. Once the membranes are broken, the barrier is gone, and risk of infection is greatly increased. This is another reason why you should avoid cervical exams. Doctors prefer to induce you so you can avoid an infection, but the truth is that you can avoid infection by keeping new bacteria from the vagina. Research shows that, compared to women who receive less than 3 cervical checks, the following is true: (276)

- o Women have 2x the risk of infection with 3-4 cervical exams
- o Women have 2.6x the risk of infection with 5-6 cervical exams
- o Women have 3.8x the risk of infection with 7-8 cervical exams
- o Women have 5x the risk of infection with more than 8 cervical exams

There are several signs that infection is developing. The American Academy of Pediatrics states that infection can be diagnosed if you have a temperature above 100.4 F and two or more of the following: (277)

- fast fetal heart rate
- fast maternal heart rate
- abdominal pain
- high white blood cell count
- foul smelling fluid

There is absolutely no correlation to term (37+ weeks) PROM and increased fetal deaths. (269)(278)

So now you are wondering what the best thing to do is if you experience PROM. Running to the hospital, a place full of germs, does nothing but set you up for opportunities for infection or medical interventions. Remember that all vaginal exams push bacteria up past the cervix, directly into contact with the baby at this point; and once you have arrived, you are on their clock.

Staying at home until labor has reached active status will allow you to ensure induction does not occur. Stay well hydrated, rest in preparation for labor, and try to enjoy the last hours before bringing your baby earthside!

If you would like to try to jumpstart labor, or your birth team is pressuring induction or transferring from a birth center, please try the natural induction methods.

Chapter 42

P.P.R.O.M.
When Your Water Breaks Too Early

PPROM is not the same as PROM. Women who have experienced their water breaking prior to the 37 week mark will tell you that it is a scary and emotional journey, as it can happen well before you are mentally ready to birth your baby.

Preterm premature rupture of the membranes (PPROM) is a true pregnancy complication. It is when your amniotic sac breaks before week 37 of pregnancy. This means that risk of infection to the uterus and baby is increased, as is your probability of delivering your baby early.

PPROM also increases the risks of other complications occurring, including: (279)

- Placental Abruption
- Prolapsed Umbilical Cord
- Miscarriage

Your labor may or may not begin on its own following PPROM, and depending on how far along you are, your labor may try to be stopped for the health and safety of your baby. If your water breaks but labor does not naturally begin, your birth team will begin a protocol to keep baby in the womb as long as possible.

PPROM is a condition that includes so many different outcomes that it is almost impossible to truly prepare a woman for experiencing it. The complication effects each baby (and mother) differently. For example, if your water breaks at 18 weeks, you are technically suffering the same condition as a mother experiencing it at 36 weeks. The outcomes, as you understand, are completely different.

Your odds of bringing home a healthy baby depend on gestational age at the time your water breaks, gestational age when labor begins, and luck – so much luck. The closer to pre-term (37 weeks) you can get, the healthier the outcome should be. Every single day inside the womb counts, and miracles happen every day.

There is no known cause for PPROM, but research has found that certain women are at a higher risk of experiencing it. Factors that may increase your chance of PPROM include: (280)(281)

- PPROM in earlier pregnancies
- Poor gut health
- Infection
- Amniocentesis
- Bleeding during the second and third trimester
- Lung disease during pregnancy
- Connective tissue disease
- Low body mass index
- Poorly developed placenta
- Smoking

As you have read, your gut health is extremely important throughout pregnancy. Again, I urge you to please consider on working toward healing your gut. Even if you think you have no real issues, there is always room for improvement.

There is no standard protocol when it comes to PPROM. Each doctor and hospital may have a different idea n proper ways to handle the complication. Doctors can decide if antibiotics should be administered and at what point they should be given. Some doctors only administer if PPROM occurs before 32 weeks, while others order them any time it occurs before 34 weeks gestation. There are some doctors who give repeat dosages of both antibiotic and steroids. This needs to be further researched, as antibiotics and steroids can potentially save the baby -- *but they can cause severe problems as well.(282)*

Remember that you have a say in your treatment plan.

Often, PPROM women are placed on bedrest if their labors can be stopped. Bed rest at home is just as safe as remaining at the hospital, so actively fight to go home. (283)

Bed rest does not mean that you cannot do other things to help prolong your pregnancy! *Studies show water intake relates directly to amniotic fluid level;* and that certain vitamins are linked to strengthening the bag of waters to prevent further rupture.

If you are placed on bed rest, consider the following:

- Increasing Vitamin C: Taking vitamin C after 14 weeks gestation is linked to preventing PPROM. (284)
- Vitamin D, Fish Oil (Omega-3), Collagen (Types 1&3), Calcium, and probiotics.
- Increase your water intake
- Exercise, even in bed.
- Eat well, avoid processed foods.
- Change your pad often to avoid bacterial growth.

Stay in a good place mentally and remember that stress can affect the outcome of labor.

Chapter 43
Preeclampsia

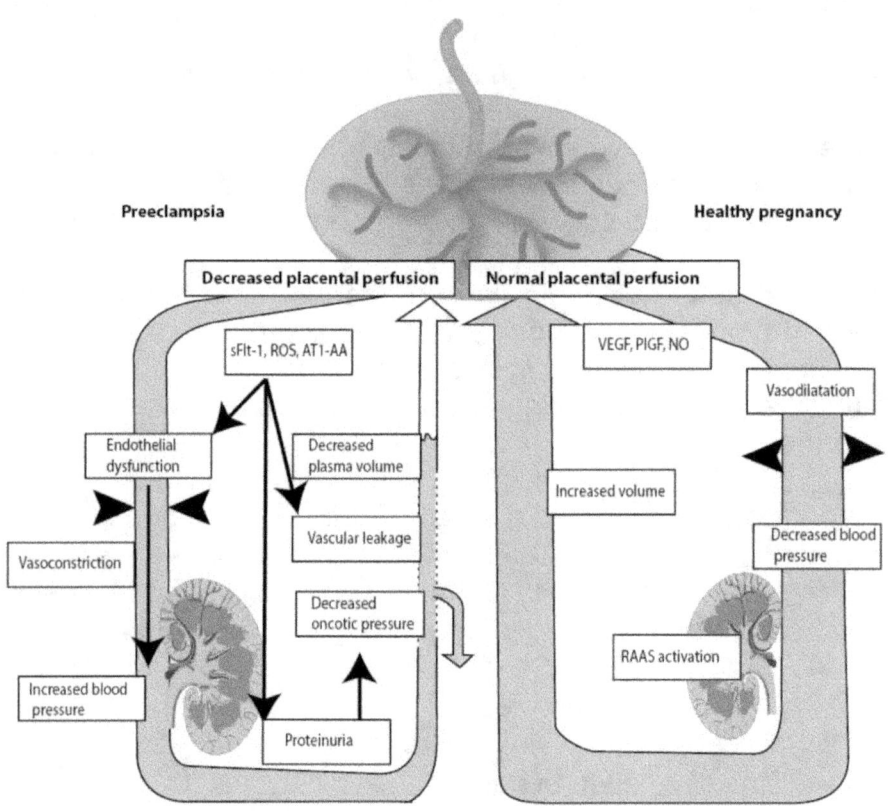

Preeclampsia is a condition that has become too common in pregnancy. It usually appears during the second half of pregnancy, typically past the 26th week of gestation or into the third trimester, although it can occur earlier. It may also occur during delivery or early postpartum. About 5-8% of pregnancies fall victim to this condition, and it can be very dangerous. (285)

If the condition is left untreated, it can turn into full eclampsia, a serious condition including seizures and possible death for mother or baby. There is absolutely no reason to take preeclampsia as a joke. Please do not ignore any signs; immediately reach out to your birth team to manage it before it gets out of hand.

According to the March of Dimes, the signs and symptoms of preeclampsia include: (285)

- High blood pressure
- Protein in the urine
- Severe headaches
- Vision problems
- Pain in the upper right belly area
- Nausea or vomiting
- Dizziness
- Sudden weight gain
- Swelling in the legs, hands, and face

Preeclampsia typically progresses fast, so if swelling is noticed, immediately take your blood pressure. There are blood pressure machines at every grocery store and pharmacy on every street corner. This swelling may not seem extreme, but if it is noticeable, it is worth checking out.

Preeclampsia is most common in your first pregnancy, and occurs more often in women with chronic high blood pressure, diabetes or a kidney disorder. The cause of preeclampsia is still unknown, but other common links include:

- Multiple gestation (twins, triplets, etc)

- Polycystic Ovarian Syndrome (PCOS)

- Family history of the disorder

- Body Mass Index (BMI) over 30%

- Over 40 years old

- Autoimmune disorders such as Lyme, rheumatoid arthritis, lupus sarcoidosis or MS.

- Previous history of preeclampsia, particularly if it occurred before the third trimester.

While science hasn't found the direct link to what is causing preeclampsia, by thoroughly reading through the research on what helps lower the risk, it is safe to say that any inflammation within the body, especially the gut, significantly increases the chances of experiencing the condition.

I have worked with many pregnant women in my practice who were trying to keep their blood pressure within the normal range so they did not experience preeclampsia, but I always have to point them to gut healing.

You know that lessening the inflammation within the gut leads to so many healing benefits, but it can also prevent preeclampsia. I know I have covered diet in detail, but the following should be included to help prevent preeclampsia from occurring.

- **Probiotics**: One study showed that daily consumption of high-quality probiotics throughout pregnancy lower the risk of preeclampsia by 39%. (286)
- **Fiber**: One study reveals that consuming 24 grams of fiber a day can reduce the risk of developing preeclampsia by 51%.(287)
- **Potassium**: Never supplement potassium on its own as it is dangerous, but a diet that includes potassium lowers pre-e risks. (288)
- **Magnesium**: Leafy green vegetables, nuts, seeds, fish, beans, lentils and avocadoes. (289)
- **B Vitamins** (methylated)
- **Vitamin D**: promotes overall health and decreases risks of developing many conditions, including pre-e.
- **Vitamin C AND E**
- **Spices**: (Tumeric, Ginger, Garlic) all have healing and anti-inflammatory properties.

- **Protein:** The Brewer's Pregnancy Diet is my first recommendation
- **Beets**: Raw Beet Juice and Beetroot are known for lowering blood pressure. (290)
- **Spirulina** (291)

Beyond diet changes, I also recommend altering lifestyle habits. Consider adding in the following:

- **Oil Pulling**: Poor dental health is linked to an increased risk of preeclampsia. Oil pulling is believed to reduce the bad bacteria that causes gum disease and other problems.
- **Sex**: Semen may help prevent preeclampsia, even when ingested through oral sex (292)
- **Exercise**: One study shows that stretching is very beneficial for mothers who have already experienced pre-e in a previous pregnancy. (293)
- **Hydration**: Proper water intake keeps the blood pressure down.

Did You Know?

If preeclampsia is diagnosed, it does not mean that you need to be admitted to the hospital and give birth immediately – although in extreme cases, this is true. Your birth team may be able to help your body better handle the pregnancy with a controlled diet, exercise plan, and plenty of rest.

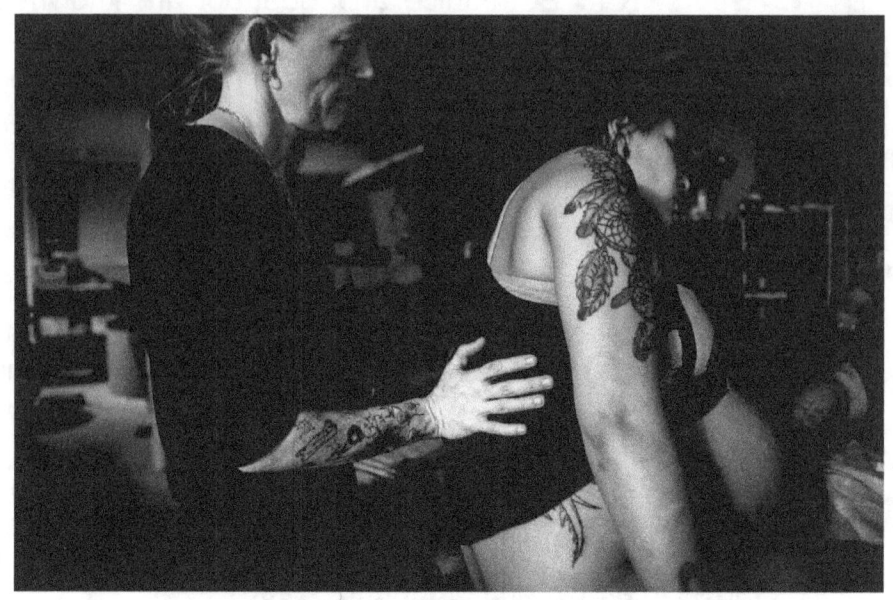

"When you go into labor you see that you are not the captain of the ship. You are the ship. There is no captain. There are only the waves."
— Karen Maezen Miller

Chapter 44
Failure to Progress

About 1/3rd of unplanned c-sections that occur in the United States are due to women "Failing to Progress" during their labor. (340) This statistic saddens me. I truly wish women would take the time to learn about pregnancy, labor and birth.

Failing to progress suggests that the woman's body is not made to give birth; that it is not dilating fast enough. How horrible to hear "You are not progressing. Your body is just not laboring well." This is *not okay*.

Failure to progress generally means a failure to wait, and a failure to allow the *woman's body to work.*

The body is not failing, it reaches a plateau. A plateau in labor refers to the timeframe that you are still consistently contracting and working hard but not showing progress through dilation. This is a naturally occurring aspect of labor and happens more often than not, and for many reasons. The most significant reason is to align baby better and ensure that both you and your baby are ready for birth. The length of this plateau is different for everyone; it can last minutes, hours, or even days (if it occurs in early labor). It is your body's way to handle labor.

It seems that most doctors give first time mothers about 20 hours of labor before declaring "failure to progress," and just 14 hours for mothers who have already given birth. If you have reached 2nd stage labor, and have pushed for over 3 hours, you may hear, "Baby is too big to come on his own." (295)

You see, doctors have adapted the mentality of 'consistent progress,' and believe labor should always look like this:

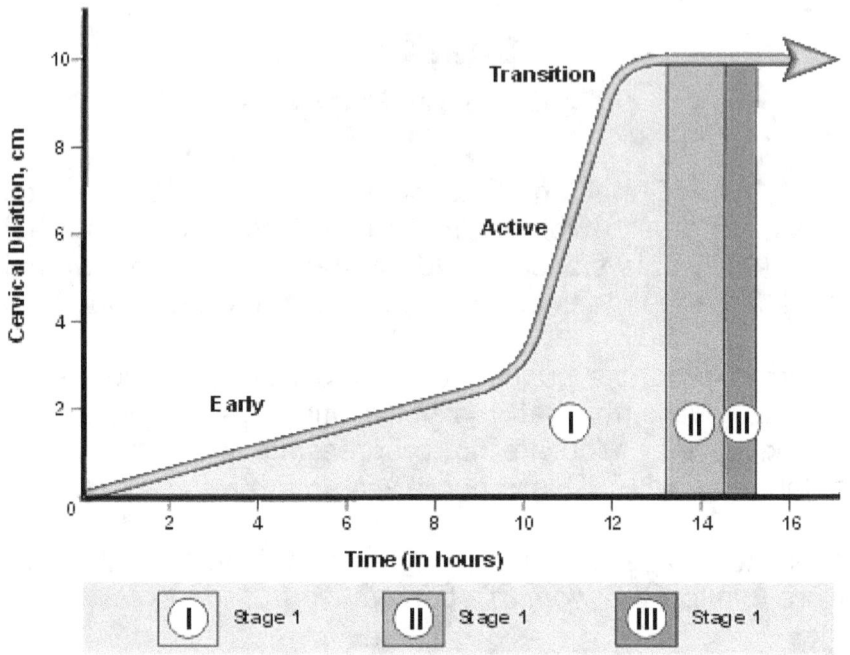

(341)

This is known as Friedman's graph, and (as you guessed) it is utterly ridiculous! Again, I am reminded of this one-size-fits all society that doesn't actually exist. Research has proven, over and over again, that the body does not labor in this pattern. With or without an epidural, the average mother does not dilate as most doctors expect. (295)(296)

The average natural, drug-free labor lasts around 15-17 hours with 6.5 of the hours being active labor. Early labor can even last days. (297)(298) I have worked with so many women whose labors lasted well over 20 hours. I am not saying that to scare you. I want you to understand that labor is natural, and your body will do what it needs to do to birth your baby. The absolute best thing you can do is have a supportive birth team who will encourage you to listen to your body.

By avoiding cervical exams all together, you will never be aware of your plateau. You will only know that you are experiencing contractions and that your body is making progress. But our society has defined labor as dilating a certain amount of centimeters over a certain period of time; not meeting this standard means your body has failed, and that you need medical help. The most common medical interventions used to 'help' women progress include: an intentional rupture of the bag of waters, Pitocin, an Epidural, and a Cesarean Section. All of which should be avoided – and can be avoided by letting the body do what it does naturally.

A c-section may be suggested if your doctor suspects that your baby may not fit through your pelvis. This is known as "CPD," and as you have read, it is extremely rare and should not be diagnosed without hours of pushing in multiple positions and an ultrasound to measure baby's head. There are extreme cases when baby is stuck and cannot be moved; these are VERY rare cases. If you believe this is happening during your labor, a doula will be your best friend, as she knows the positions to move you in to help birth baby in the position he seems to be stuck. Extreme cases are need for surgical intervention.

My co-author and I have been a part of the birthing community for many years and we have witnessed, discussed, read about, and experienced plateau in labor. We agree that the reasoning behind a plateau can be different for every birthing mother, but that the most common explanations of needing more time include:

Baby's Position and Achieving Better Alignment. Your baby may be "Sunny-Side Up" (OP position), have a hand by his face, or is just in a funky position. The extra time and contractions may be needed for a better manipulation of his body down the birth canal.

Massaging Baby. Contractions may not be comfortable for you, but they act as a massage to the baby. This massage stimulates the nervous system and lungs, preparing them both for entering the world.

Pelvic Changes. Your pelvis softens as it opens. Laboring in different positions can help in this process, but it may just take time and extra contractions.

Antibodies. The breasts form all immunities necessary to protect the baby against your birthing environment after birth while you are in labor. (299) Sometimes, the breasts need more time to produce these antibodies. The process should not be rushed.

It's Psychological. Emotions, fears, stress, anxiety, anything you are holding on to can cause you to plateau longer than needed. Letting go and giving into your labor, even changing positions and moving can help. The same can be said for your baby! Think of all the new emotions and changes happening to your baby during labor. He could possibly need time to process the entire journey.

Dilation means nothing, but the urge to push means everything. You can be at 3 cm for 10 hours of labor and dilate from 3-10cm in 30 minutes. You could plateau at 8cm for 5 hours and be ready to give up when the urge to push overwhelms you. There is no exact science to birthing your baby. Listening to your body is the best plan. Make sure you are never lying on your back, as your body has to fight gravity.

Did You Know?

Induction and medical interventions can lead to a true "Failure to Progress," but not because the baby is stuck, instead because the baby *was not ready to be born yet*. Allowing your labor to be induced or medically altered, you increase the risk of labor not going as you may have wanted.

Chapter 45
Suctioning at Birth

Once baby is born, but before he is placed on your chest, some doctors still practice the outdated procedure of suctioning the airways. Clinical guidelines no longer recommend suctioning a baby's airways *'unless they are unresponsive, floppy and require resuscitation.'* Even then, suctioning should be done with a laryngoscope and not a bulb.(300)

Most birth teams have let go of this procedure, but yet so many perform it due to habit. It is important to discuss it with your doctor or midwife, as there are many dangers linked to suctioning at birth.

There is a natural 'Fetal Heimlich Maneuver' that occurs as the baby is born. If you have the chance to watch natural birth videos, look closely as the head surfaces and rotates. You will notice fluid be expelled through the mouth and nose. It happens in the blink of an eye, but it is such an amazing process. It occurs when the intact perineum squeezes his breastbone as he passes through. This pushes amniotic fluid out of his esophagus and mouth naturally, leaving no need to be suctioned. The act of suctioning can actually cause your baby to receive less oxygen than is optimal.

It is normal (and natural) for your baby to work fluid out as he transitions over to using his own lungs to breathe. It is not natural or normal for a baby to have a bulb syringe gag him in the throat in the first moments of his life.

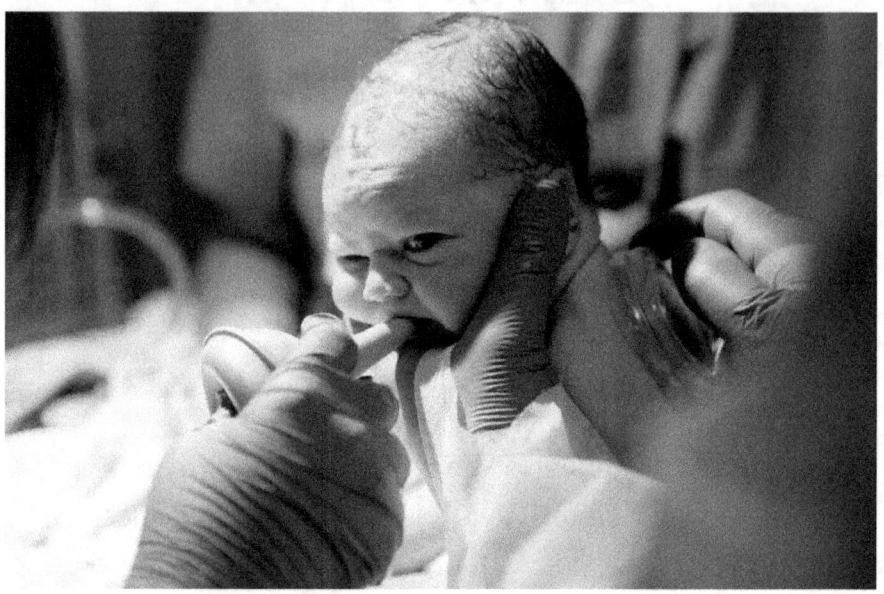

Suctioning can truly hurt your baby, physically and emotionally. There are so many reasons that I suggest you try to avoid allowing this at your baby's birth (and why you should not practice it throughout his infancy).

Suctioning your baby's airways can cause: (301)

- Damage to your breastfeeding relationship (302)
- Increase risk of MAS due to causing your baby to inhale deeply, which is what you want to avoid

- Vagal Bradycardia: the lowering of your baby's heart rate for up to 20 minutes (303)
- Trauma to mucous membranes
- Laryngospasm
- Cardiac Dysrhythmias
- Edema
- Tachycardia
- Emotional Distress
- Bronchospasm
- Cardiac Arrest

Some newborns take longer to transition earthside than others. Hearing the gurgling sound at birth of a brand new baby can be scary, but it is normal. Let your baby work it out.

Did You Know?

The latest research now shows that babies who have their faces wiped during birth and immediately after have a clinical outcome that is exactly the same as those who are suctioned, but without any of the risk factors. (304)

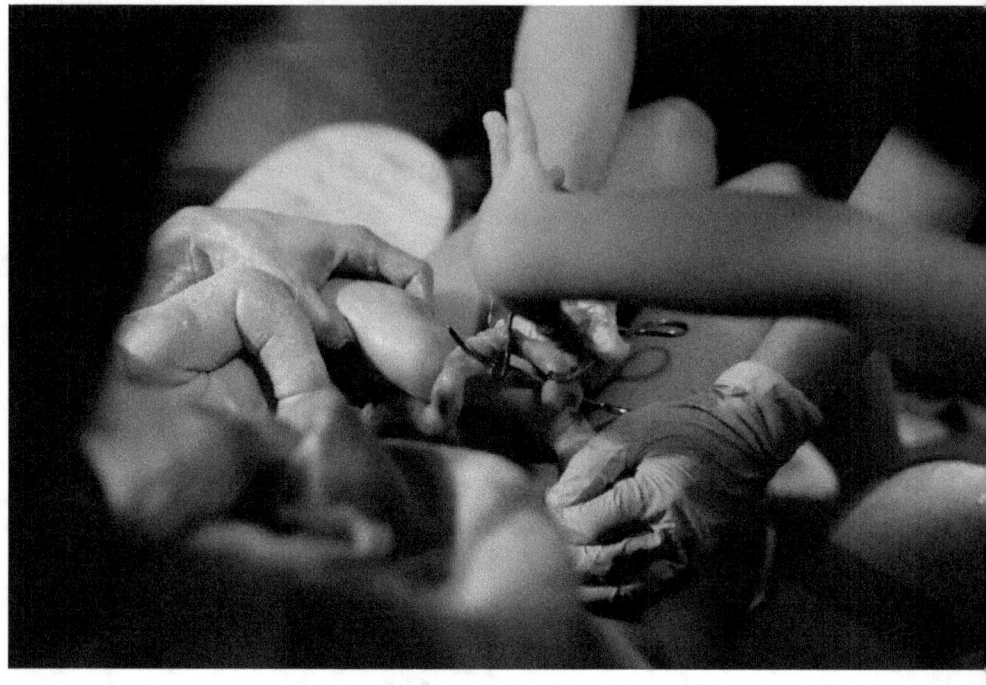

(cutting of the umbilical cord)

"The life of a mother is the life of a child. You are two blossoms on the same branch." - Karen Maezen Miller

Chapter 46
Delayed Cord Clamping
Let it Pulse

Just like the placenta, the umbilical cord is severely underestimated. At least science has convinced people on the valuable blood that lies within it, but yet, so many don't put two and two together. That amazing cord blood that does so many wonderful things should be *INSIDE* the baby that was connected to it in the womb.

Most women don't look at the umbilical cord in detail after giving birth; and they are missing out on something fascinating. This cord, with the help of the placenta, is what provided all nutrients to your baby in utero. It was responsible for transporting everything to and from you and your baby.

Hopefully, your birth team practices delayed cord clamping and it will not be something you have to fight for – but even if it is part of their birth protocol, taking the time to watch it happen will help you understand just why it's so important.

A series of events take place as your baby comes earthside, and they happen quicker than you would be able to witness them. However, the ACOG and March of Dimes both stress the importance of having patience during this period. There should be no rush, as the placenta, umbilical cord, and baby still have work to perform together – important work.

If you take nothing else away from this book, take this: Labor and birth are natural. They deserve your trust and patience -and belief that there is a reason, a purpose for each ordinary step of bringing a healthy baby into this world.

In most hospital deliveries, there is little to no delay, instead

287

there is almost a rush to cut the umbilical cord, which can cause a lot of immediate issues for your baby.

While in utero, your baby has around a 60% oxygen saturation due to the mix of fresh blood from the placenta and the de-oxygenated blood moving toward his heart. This is a much lower saturation level than he will experience outside of the womb at 95-98%. When your baby is born, his body must transfer from receiving oxygen from the placenta to his lungs. His lungs will expand, but to do so properly, they require a rush of blood from the umbilical cord. The cord also helps transition your baby to this new environment, as it slowly transports the last of the mixed blood from the placenta. (305) (306)

At birth, your baby's lungs are still quite restrained, causing a high amount of pressure within his circulatory system. Remember that his lungs are filled with fluid when he is in the womb, which forces the blood to be limited within the vessels of the lungs. This high pressure condition can be quite taxing, but because the placenta houses very little pressure, your baby's blood would flow back to it. This means that the placenta is holding a significant amount of the blood that is meant to be in your baby. Allowing the cord to pulse until completion allows for approximately 30% more blood volume to enter your baby.

Did You Know?

Without delayed cord clamping, your baby does not receive the rush of blood needed to prevent a drastic drop in blood pressure - as his lungs may fail to open properly. Most full-term babies will have enough blood to prevent brain damage, but immediate cord clamping can still leave them weak. Premature babies are severely in need of this cord blood.

Immediate cord clamping can lead to: (307)(308) (309)(310)

- Infant anemia (resulting in cognitive deficits)
- Autism
- Cerebral Palsy
- Anemia
- Learning disorders and mental deficiency
- Brain hemorrhage
- Brain damage
- Lung damage
- Breathing problems
- Hypotension
- Hypovolemia
- Behavioral disorders
- Respiratory distress

Delayed cord clamping means not cutting the umbilical cord after birth until all of the blood has finished pulsing through it. Trust me, you'll know when it has finished. The majority of the blood will transfer in the first 5-15 minutes after birth. Your baby's heart beat causes the cord to pulsate until the placental circulation has completed. Gravity plays a huge rule in the amount of blood transferred, and holding your baby skin-to-skin will help the process. (311)

The umbilical cord clamps naturally once all the blood has been transferred to your baby; it will stop pulsing and turn white after the transfer is complete.

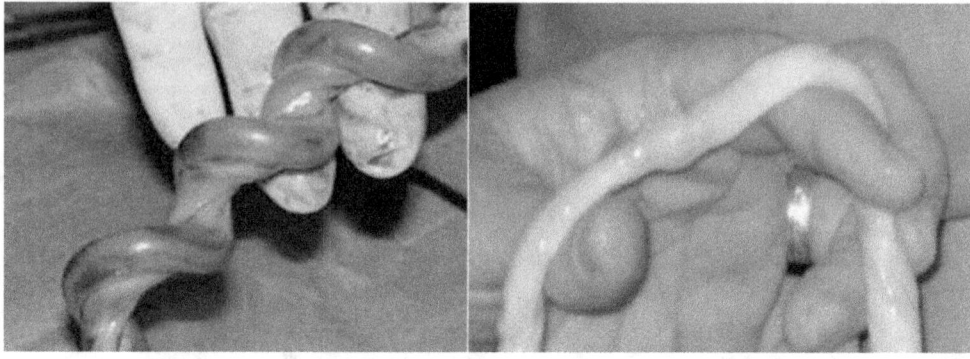

http://www.vaccinationinformationnetwork.com/cord-clamping-and-stem-cell-collection-by-hilary-butler/

Choosing to allow your baby's cord to pulse allows for the following: (312)(313)(314)(315) (316)

- Decreased frequency of Iron Deficiency Anemia
- Improved Neurodevelopment
- Improved systemic blood pressure
- Improved urine output
- Improved cardiac function
- Decreased chance of sepsis
- Reduced need for blood transfusions
- Decreased risk of intraventricular hemorrhage
- Increased red cell formations
- Reduced risk of immediate resuscitation

There is rarely a situation in which delayed cord clamping is not beneficial. Delayed cord clamping is especially beneficial in helping a baby who is born with a cord around the neck, or born prematurely, or with breathing difficulties. (317) If the baby is not breathing when they're born, allowing the cord to continue pulsing means that they're still receiving oxygen through the cord.

Delayed cord clamping can even take pace in the OR during

a C-section. But there are few instances in which it may not be safe for the cord to be left intact. These include: (311)

- Placental abruption
- Cord damage
- Cord prolapse
- Rare blood conditions

Even delaying for as few as 3 minutes can be beneficial to your baby. It can mean having a child with higher social and neurodevelopmental abilities. The World Health Organization stance is " *Delayed umbilical cord clamping (not earlier than 1 min after birth) is recommended for improved maternal and infant health and nutrition outcomes.*"(318) It may seem like such a small battle, almost not worth fighting, but I urge you to fight this one. No matter your birth plan or labor experience goes, delaying the cord clamping should rank high or your priority list.

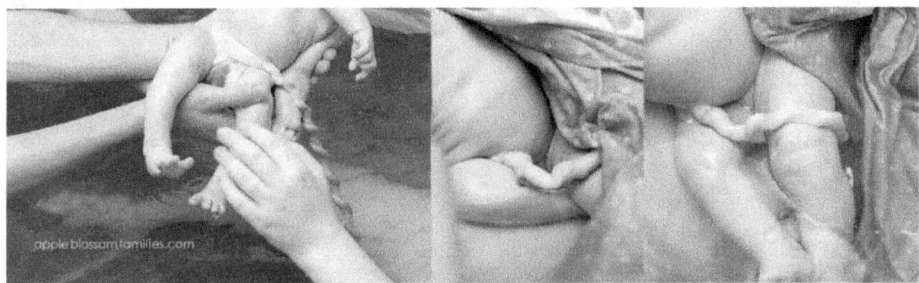

The image is 45 *seconds* post birth, 12 minutes post birth and 23 minutes post birth, retrospectively. (Photo: Appleblossomfamilies.com)

Chapter 47
Unneeded Eye Ointment

It's such a shame that our culture interferes so much with pregnancy and birth, but in truth, that is just the beginning. Once your baby is born, that is when so many interventions are thrown at you – but you have a choice. It is your right to accept or deny any or all of these practices. Remember how natural and normal it is for us to conceive, grow, labor, and birth a baby; there is no reason that, within moments of being born, that perfectly healthy being needs intervention. It is time for us to spread our wanting for hands-off pregnancy, birth, and newborn care. This is not a 'crunchy' way of thinking, but instead it is the safest, healthiest and most natural way to bring new life to the world.

In the late 1800's, silver nitrate was used in newborn's eyes to prevent blindness, but it irritated and caused many problems. Years later, doctors found that placing erythromycin antibiotic ointment in a newborn's eyes immediately after birth would prevent gonorrhea, chlamydia, and syphilis from blinding the baby. This had much fewer side effects than the silver nitrate, and produced good results. (319)

Here we are, over 100 years later and the outdated practice is still performed on the eyes of every single newborn whose parents do not know that they can deny it. The ointment is lined inside the lower eyelids within the first 2 hours of life; it is done quickly and most often without talking to the parents about it first. So you may need to speak up – or require all newborn care/procedures be done while your baby is skin-to-skin with you.

I understand that this use to save babies from becoming blind, but our world is not the same as it was 100 years ago. Back then, Ophthalmia Neonatorum (ON) affects 10% of all babies and caused blindness to 3% of those affected. (This means

0.3% of newborns were truly affected) 135 years later we actually have specific medicine to treat ON if it is contracted during birth. This defeats the entire purpose of using the antibiotic ointment on all the eyes of all the babies. So why is it still happening? I believe that it is purely habit, tradition, and failure to adapt and change. (320)

Your baby is born with vision that reaches about 12", the same distance from your breast to your face. Coincidence? No. Your baby is supposed to be breastfeeding and learning your face right now. The eye ointment completely impedes this from happening. The very important visual bonding cannot take place, as the ointment blurs everything for the first day of life. Not only is bonding affected, but there are risks of reactions to the antibiotic and disruption of the healthy gut flora.

If you have an active STD during labor and birth, you should talk with your birth team about other options, but if you are healthy there is absolutely no need to consent to this procedure.

Canadian pediatricians have been trying to eliminate the application of the antibiotic; these doctors have confirmed that the ointment does not actually work. (321) It does not treat most strains of gonorrhea or chlamydia, the very conditions that would lead to blindness. (322)

The lesson that you should take away from this: INFORMED CONSENT.

Chapter 48
Vitamin K and Your Options

Besides eye ointment, Vitamin K is also routinely given at birth, often without speaking to the parents first. I personally believe that it is not needed immediately, but I respect your decision either way needs to be discussed beforehand. However, know that the synthetic version given by most birth workers is not natural. There are other options available.

Vitamin K is necessary for normal blood clotting in adults and children, but newborns are different. Newborns are not born with, what has been deemed, 'sufficient' amounts of the vitamin. This alone makes me question the need of an intervention. If all babies are born with little Vitamin K, it may be because that is what is meant to be. Nature may have a purpose to this.

It is quite rare, but you should know that Vitamin K deficiency can lead to a serious bleeding disorder within the first week of life. This disorder, called Hemorrhagic Disease of the Newborn (HDN) is an internal bleeding that happens in the brain and other organs, and can lead to injury or death. Preventing this should of course be of concern, but instead of injecting all newborns, perhaps risk factors and observation and individualized care should take place.

HDN may affect 0.25% of infants, but there are several risk factors linked to the disorder: (323)

- Low birth weight
- Preterm delivery
- A forceps or vacuum extraction delivery
- Medications taken while pregnant
- Precipitous or prodromal labor
- C-section
- Undiagnosed liver problems
- Hepatitis

- Cystic fibrosis
- Celiac disease
- Alpha – 1-antitrypsin deficiency
- Other genetic disorders

Vitamin K Deficiency Bleeding (VKDB) can occur within 3 different timeframes: (323)(324)

- Early Onset occurs in the first 24 hours of life and is linked to mothers who took medicines that interfere with Vitamin K.
- Classical VKDB occurs between days 2-7 (days 2-3 are most common) when vitamin K levels are at their lowest.
- Late Onset occurs after day 7, typically during weeks 3-8.

Circumcisions performed within the first few days of life have contributed to making Vitamin K injections common. Receiving the shot lowers the risk of excessive bleeding from the circumcision. Yes, there is a chance your son could bleed to death (among so many other lifelong problems or side effects) from receiving a circumcision. There are no actual health benefits, and the cosmetic surgery (as insurance companies have labeled it) should be avoided.

Vitamin K levels rise naturally within your baby. This occurs at the same pace – over the first week - as the liver fully developing and being able to detoxify his body. Un-metabolized Vitamin K (the synthetic dose injected) does not show up in the urine, which is cause for concern because vitamin K is a fat soluble vitamin and can accumulate in body tissue.

Your baby's natural levels will peak around day 8 of life. Research shows that this is related to the bacteria in the newborn's gut.(325) (Again, I urge you to work on healing and having a healthy gut while pregnant. There is so much riding on your baby's gut development.)

There are 2 forms of Vitamin K, K1 and K2. K2 is transported in high amounts through the placenta, increasing more so in the third trimester. K1 is not noticeably passed to the baby while in utero, but this should not be flagged as a problem, as it naturally occurs this way. (326)

The vitamin K that is passed through your breastmilk is the natural version of the vitamin and will be more optimally absorbed by your baby. So you may want to consider (and I highly recommend) consuming a natural vitamin K through diet or supplement while breastfeeding. Research shows that the amount of Vitamin K in breastmilk changes as the baby grows, starting with a higher amount in the first few days and lessening over time. Colostrum, the first milk you produce, contains significantly higher levels of Vitamin K than your mature milk. So you should breastfeed within the first hour after birth and as often as your baby will nurse in those first few days. (327)(328)

Accepting the synthetic Vitamin K injection (even the preservative-free version) at birth places your baby at risk for: (329)

- Gasping Syndrome in premature infants
- Severe or fatal allergic reactions (hives, swelling, breathing trouble)
- Bleeding or bruising at injection site
- Death
- Hyperbilirubinemia
- Pain: Not only do infants feel pain, but the earlier they experience it, the more damaging and longer lasting the psychological effects. (331)

Directly from the manufacturer's insert: (329)

"Severe reactions, including fatalities, have occurred during and immediately after INTRAVENOUS injection of phytonadione, even when precautions have been taken to dilute the phytonadione and to avoid rapid infusion. Severe reactions, including fatalities, have also been reported following INTRAMUSCULAR administration. Typically these severe reactions have resembled hypersensitivity or anaphylaxis, including shock and cardiac and/or respiratory arrest."

The amount of vitamin K in the injection is significantly higher than your baby's vitamin K level at birth. I feel as though I am always talking to my patience about the importance of correctly dosing their vitamins. This should be no exception.

Educating yourself on your options is important. While you can choose to deny the intervention, you may also decide to opt for supplementing either yourself (to be passed through your breastmilk) or your baby orally.

Chapter 49
Planning a Homebirth

As you have gathered, laboring and birthing in your home environment is not only safe, but best for a healthy mom and baby. I understand if you would rather birth in a birth center, as that too is a place of peacefulness and happiness. The hospital can make for a challenging location to have a peaceful birth, but it can be done.

I do hope that you at least consider birthing at home.

A recent study confirms that among low-risk women, planned home births result in low rates of interventions without an increase in adverse outcomes for mothers and babies. This means that you are more likely to have the birth you desire, free of interventions, if you birth at home with a midwife. (331)

The first step in a successful home birth is having both you and your partner on board. This may take sitting down with a midwife and asking a long list of questions before you are comfortable. When you begin meeting midwives (yes, plural. I believe you should shop around and find the one you most connect with), consider asking some of the following questions:

About her:
- How many births have you attended?
- How long have you been a midwife?
- Are you licensed to practice in this state?
- Are you certified in neonatal resuscitation?
- How many births do you commit to attending per month?
- Have you missed a birth? Why?
- Do you take insurance?

About birth:
- What would risk me out of a home birth?
- What is your transfer rate?
- What is your transfer plan? Which hospital would we go to?
- Under what circumstances would you recommend a transfer?
- Will you deliver a breech baby?
- What is my window of time to deliver: 37-42 weeks?
- What testing do you recommend?
- Who attends the birth with you?
- What medications do you carry with you to births?
- What is your personal philosophy on birth?

When I was writing *Crunchy Mom's,* I asked one of my favorite homebirth midwives, Karen Webster,CPM,LM who has attended over 1,000 births since 1979, what would she like a family to know about home birth when they are not sure about having a baby at home. Mrs. Webster explains, " I remind them that births have only taken place in hospitals with OB's less than 100 years. Birthing in the hospital is <u>experimental</u>, meaning the odds of having a normal low to no intervention birth in a hospital are not good even if you are a healthy woman. The odds of having a surgical birth or Cesarean are roughly 1 in 3. Epidural rates are at roughly 85% depending on the hospital. Those looking to have a VBAC (vaginal birth after Cesarean) your odds are 8-11% should your hospital allow it to be done.

In other countries, Europe, UK and Canada, midwives are the primary caregiver for most healthy pregnant women. OB's and physicians are utilized when there are complications during pregnancy."

Mrs. Webster encourages families to also do their homework and to ask many questions like we have stated above. She also wants you to envision conceiving a child in a hospital setting with monitors, all the personnel in and out of the room, and constant nurses taking vital signs.

"Birth is an a extension of the very intimate act of conceiving a child, and by nature, sexual, and sacred."- Karen Webster, CPM, LM, WomenWise Midwifery

After you have asked all of your questions, and you feel comfortable with your decision, the fun part starts! You get to plan a homebirth! Register for a natural birthing class. The Bradley Method, Hypnobirthing, Birthing From Within, and other Independent Birth Classes will all serve you well.

So, having a strong support system can play a huge role in a successful and peaceful homebirth. Spend time telling your friends and family about your choice, but ask them to keep negative feelings away. You can keep them feeling included by asking them to light a candle for you once labor starts. It symbolizes positive prayers and thoughts for a peaceful birth.

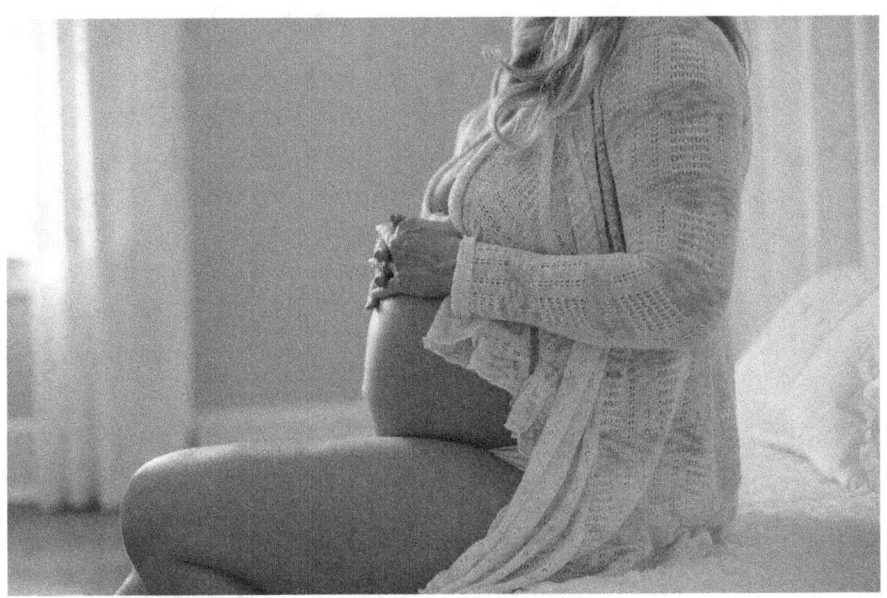

"If women lose the right to say where and how they birth their children, then they will have lost something that's as dear to life as breathing."
— Ami McKay, The Birth House

Chapter 50
Writing your birth plan

There is a reason I have saved this chapter until the end of the book; you see, my hope is for you to have truly read and learned about everything I wanted to share. Once you have digested it all, it is time to truly look at your pregnancy and upcoming labor. It is time to set your priorities and create your birth plan.

A birth plan is not just about bringing your baby into the world safely. It is about so much more; the entire journey of labor and birth. Your birth plan is a culmination of your research; a brief proposal of what you would like, how things should be handled, and how you deserve to be treated.

Before writing your birth plan, tour your birthing facility and schedule a time to talk with your doctor, or midwife. You cannot begin this until all of your questions are answered. You need to know what the standard of care is from the moment you enter the facility until the second you are wheeled out. (Are you allowed to walk out? -simple questions like that need to be asked too!)

Once you have a basic timeline of events, you can dig into the research and figure out your priorities. I have yet to ever see two identical birth plans.

The easier the plan is to read, the higher the chances are that it will be read. Remember not to include why you are asking for these things, that does not matter.

The following is a sample birth plan. Yours will be your own, but feel free to start here and alter as you like. It is based on a natural hospital birth without medical intervention. Remember, you may not agree with this plan, but that's the beauty of it – you get to make your own!

Sample Birth Plan

I would like to have an unmedicated vaginal birth and would like your help in accomplishing it. If anything occurs in which interventions may be needed, please help us to continue on the most natural path possible, and allow us the time to make decisions.

In case of emergency, save both mother and baby in any way possible.

*There will be a photographer with us, and we want her with us in all situations.

Before Labor

- No cervical checks
- I would like to let labor begin naturally, even past my due date.
- PROM: I would like 48-72 hours before any interventions are suggested. I agree to have my fluid levels monitored after 24 hours.

Early Labor

- I want the ability to leave if labor is still early, even if my water has broken.
- GBS: I deny antibiotics and will watch for signs of illness after birth.
- I would prefer no heparin lock, but will compromise if an IV will not be attached.

Active Labor

- DO NOT OFFER PAIN MANAGEMENT MEDICATIONS.
- My partner will stay with me at all times and be included in all discussions.
- I would like a peaceful, environment with few interruptions.
- I would like stand, move and walk freely.
- I will eat and drink throughout labor.
- I would like access to the birthing tub.
- No cervical checks unless requested.
- Do not break my water.
- No electronic fetal monitoring, internal monitoring, or wireless monitoring. If continuous monitoring is needed, I will allow wireless monitoring.

2nd Stage Labor

- No episiotomy unless I am naturally tearing toward my clitoris.
- No instrumental interventions (forceps or vacuum)
- Please do not instruct my pushing.
- I would like access to the squat bar and birth stool.
- I would like to 'catch' my baby, or have my partner catch the baby.
- My partner will announce the baby's gender.
- Baby will immediately be placed skin to skin on my chest.
- We will let the umbilical cord pulse to completion before clamping.

3rd Stage Labor

- No medical interventions to birth the placenta.
- Placenta will be kept in the provided cooler

C-Section

- A c-section will only be performed once all options have been exhausted and it is a medical emergency.
- My partner will remain with me throughout the procedure.
- No general anesthesia. I would like to have feeling and the ability to move my arms.
- I would like to be included in the birth conversation during surgery.
- Baby will be placed directly on my chest (if possible) with the umbilical cord and placenta still attached.
- Take extreme care with incision and sutures to support a future VBAC and more pregnancies.

Following Birth

- Myself, my partner or my child will cut the cord after it has finished pulsing.
- No separation from baby. Anything needed can be done with baby on my chest.
- In an emergency, my partner will stay with the baby.
- Breastfeeding will be attempted before any newborn procedures.
- Vernix will be rubbed into the baby's skin
- Do not bathe (or wipe) baby

- We will have a golden hour of bonding
- No Vitamin K injection
- No antibiotic eye ointment
- NO VACCINES: I decline the hepB vaccine and any other vaccines or injections offered.
- DO NOT CIRCUMSIZE if baby is a boy (or a girl).
- No formula.
- No Bottles.
- No pacifiers.
- I would like a lactation consultant to be available as soon after delivery as possible.

A birth plan is not written in stone. No matter what though, YOU SHOULD NEVER BE PUSHED OR TALKED INTO ANYTHING. If situations arise, take the time to talk about your options, risks, and make informed decisions.

"If I had my life to live over, instead of wishing away nine months of pregnancy, I'd have cherished every moment and realized that the wonderment growing inside me was the only chance in life to assist God in a miracle." - Irma Bombeck

ABOUT THE AUTHORS

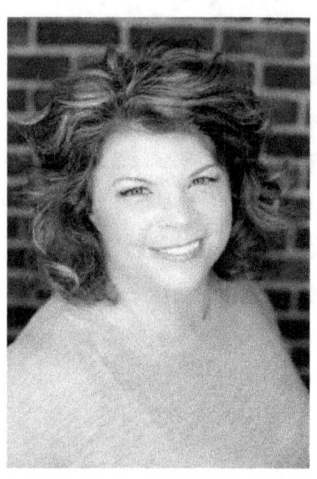

Dr. Brenda Fairchild is one of the leading chiropractors in pregnancy and pediatrics and has a practice dedicated to the health and wellbeing of women and children. Dr. Brenda is so passionate about what she does, she is continuously educating herself not only in the chiropractic field, but as well as midwifery, pediatrics, and functional medicine. She has an amazing family from which her passion of pregnancy and pediatrics came about. It was through her own pregnancy that she found her calling which Madelyn Jaymes.

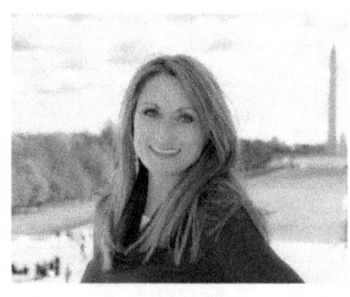

Elizabeth MacDonald holds a degree in Exercise Physiology, is a research writer, a pre/postnatal Exercise Specialist and a natural childbirth educator. She enjoys finding a holistic solution to a medical problem, and believes strongly in trusting the woman's body to grow and birth her baby. Elizabeth is a home birthing mother to four, with a supportive husband whom she loves passionately. Her family drives her desire to research, and inspires her to constantly become a better person.

Photo Credits Throughout Book!

The Amazing Cover by:

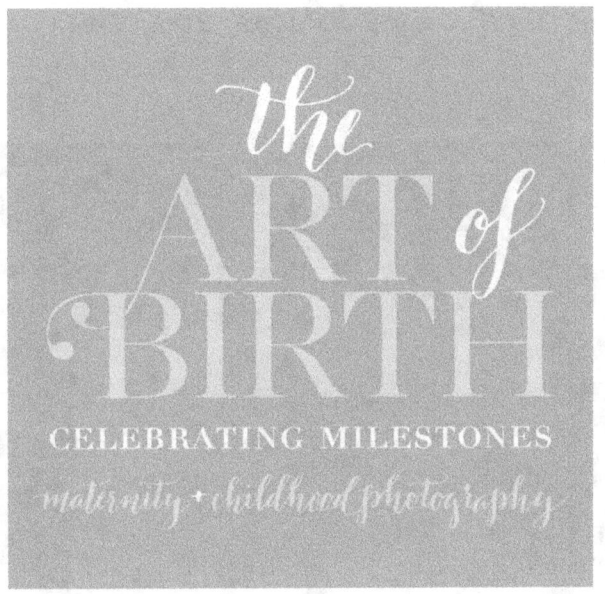

Pictures of Dr. Brenda in office by:

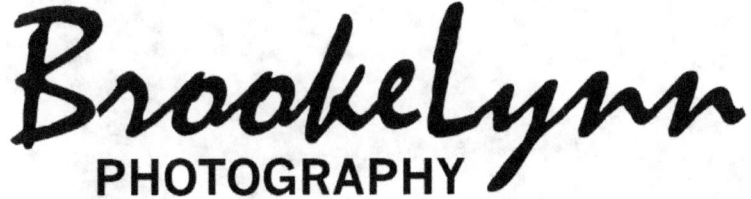

Make sure you have Dr. Brenda's bestselling first book on raising a healthy child naturally. You will find natural remedies on helping to keep you child well to constipation, colic, headaches, and reflux.

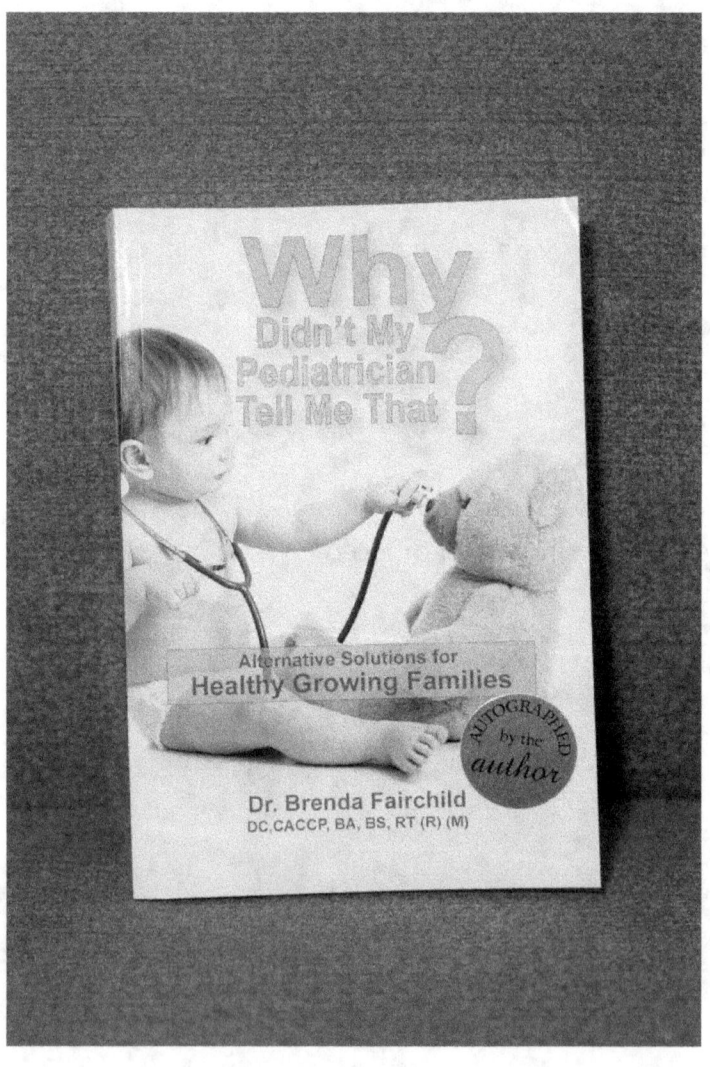

Bibliography

1. Office on Women's Health Organization.
    www.womenshealth.gov
2. Pahuja, M. 18-20 Week Screening Pregnancy
    Ultrasound. Inside Radiology. The Royal Australian
    and New Zealand College of Radiologists.
    http://www.insideradiology.com.au/pages/view.php?T
    _id=68#.V7L-Rzjgapp
3. American Congress of Obstetricians and
    Gynecologists. Oct. 22, 2013.
    http://www.acog.org/About-ACOG/News-Room/News-
    Releases/2013/Ob-Gyns-Redefine-Meaning-of-Term-
    Pregnancy
4. Borggren, Cara. Pregnancy and chiropractic: a
    narrative review of the literature. Journal of
    Chiropractic Medicine. June 2007 Volume 6, Issue 2,
    Pages 70–74.
5. International Chiropractic Pediatric Association.
    About the Webster Technique.
    http://icpa4kids.com/about/webster_technique.htm
6. Diakow PR, Gadsby TA, Gadsby JB, Gleddie JG,
    Leprich DJ, Scales AM. 1991 (Feb). Back pain during
    pregnancy and labor. J Manipulative Physiol Ther. 14
    (2): 116-118
7. Mercola, Joseph. Top Foods to Eat When You're
    Pregnant. Nov.02, 2015.
    http://articles.mercola.com/sites/articles/archive/2015/
    11/02/top-pregnancy-foods.aspx
8. Carmichael SL, Yang W, Feldkamp ML, Munger RG,
    Siega-Riz AM, Botto LD, Shaw G; National Birth
    Defects Prevention Study. Reduced risks of neural

tube defects and orofacial clefts with higher diet quality. Arch Pediatr Adolesc Med. 2012 Feb;166(2):121-6

9. Imdad, A. Bhutta, Z. Effect of balanced protein energy supplementation during pregnancy on birth outcomes. BMC Public Health. 2011; 11(Suppl 3): S17. Published online 2011 Apr 13.

10. Jimenez, E. Marin, M. Martin, R. et al. Is meconium from healthy newborns actually sterile? Research in Microbiology Volume 159, Issue 3, April 2008, Pages 187–193

11. Matamoros, S. Gras-Leguen, C. Le Vacon, F. Potel, G. de La Cochetiere, MF. Development of intestinal microbiota in infants and its impact on health. Trends Microbiol. 2013 Apr;21(4):167-73

12. Prince, AL. Antony, KM. Ma, J. Aagaard, KM. The microbiome and development: a mother's perspective. Semin Reprod Med. 2014 Jan;32(1):14-22

13. Rautava, S. Collado, M.C. Salminen, S.. Isolauri, E. Probiotics Modulate Host-Microbe Interaction in the Placenta and Fetal Gut: A Randomized, Double-Blind, Placebo-Controlled Trial. Neonatology 2012;102:178–184

14. Koren, O. Goodrich, J. Cullender, T. et al. Host Remodeling of the Gut Microbiome and Metabolic Changes during Pregnancy. Cell. Volume 150, Issue 3, p470–480, 3 August 2012

15. Stuefer S, Moncayo H, Moncayo R. The role of magnesium and thyroid function in early pregnancy after in-vitro fertilization (IVF): New aspects in endocrine physiology. BBA Clinical. 2015 Mar 5;3:196-204

16. Moyer, M. Gut Bacteria May Play a Role in Autism. Scientific American. Sept. 1, 2014

17. Hsiao,E. McBride, S. Hsien, S. et al. The microbiota modulates gut physiology and behavioral

abnormalities associated with autism. Cell. 2013 Dec 19; 155(7): 1451–1463.

18. Backhed, F. Roswall, J. et al. Dynamics and Stabilization of the Human Gut Microbiome during the First Year of Life. Cell Host and Microbe. Volume 17, Issue 5, p690–703, 13 May 2015

19. Mercola, Joseph. The Importance of Reducing Your Toxic Burden When Planning to Start a Family. December 27, 2014. http://articles.mercola.com/sites/articles/archive/2014/12/27/seeding-baby-microbiome.aspx#_edn7

20. WebMD. Retailers Accused of Selling Fake Supplements. Feb.3, 2015. http://www.webmd.com/vitamins-and-supplements/news/20150203/retailers-fake-supplements

21. Kim, Young-In. Folic Acid Supplementation and Cancer Risk: Point. Cancer Epidemiol Biomarkers Prev September 2008 17; 2220

22. Designs for Health. Folic Acid vs. Folate: Part I. Nov 28, 2011. http://blog.designsforhealth.com/blog/bid/115121/Folic-Acid-vs-Folate-Part-I

23. Klemens, CM. Berman, DR. Mozurkewich, EL. The effect of perinatal omega-3 fatty acid supplementation on inflammatory markers and allergic diseases: a systematic review. BJOG: An International Journal of Obstetrics and Gynaecology. 2011 Jul;118(8):916-25

24. American Pregnancy Association. Omega-3 Fish Oil and Pregnancy. http://americanpregnancy.org/pregnancy-health/omega-3-fish-oil/

25. American Congress of Obstetricians and Gynecologists. August 2009. Committee on Ethics. Informed Consent. http://www.acog.org/Resources-

And-Publications/Committee-Opinions/Committee-on-Ethics/Informed-Consent

26. Imdad, A. Bhutta, Z. Effect of balanced protein energy supplementation during pregnancy on birth outcomes. BioMed Central public health. 2011.

27. Hofmeyr, GJ et al. Low-dose calcium supplementation for preventing pre-eclampsia: a systematic review and commentary. BJOG. 2014 Jul; 121(8): 951–957.

28. Yan, J. et al. Maternal choline supplementation programs greater activity of the phosphatidylethanolamine N-methyltransferase (PEMT) pathway in adult Ts65Dn trisomic mice. The Journal of the Federation of American Societies for Experimental Biology. 2014 Oct; 28(10): 4312–4323.

29. Morse, N. Benefits of Docosahexaenoic Acid, Folic Acid, Vitamin D and Iodine on Foetal and Infant Brain Development and Function Following Maternal Supplementation during Pregnancy and Lactation. Nutrients. 2012 Jul; 4(7): 799–840.

30. Tam,C. O'connor, D. Koren, G. Circulating Unmetabolized Folic Acid: Relationship to Folate Status and Effect of Supplementation. Obstetrics and Gynecology International. 2012; 2012: 485179.

31. Yarrington, C. Pearce, E. Iodine and Pregnancy. Journal of Thyroid Research. June 13,2011.

32. Pena-Rosas, J. et al. Daily oral iron supplementation during pregnancy. Cochrane Database Syst Rev. 2012; 12: CD004736.

33. Kelly, T. Gu, D. et al. Maternal History of Hypertension and Blood Pressure Response to Potassium Intake. The GenSalt Study. American Journal of Epidemiology. 2012 Oct 1; 176(Suppl 7): S55–S63.

34. Meharaban, Z. et al. Restless Legs Syndrome During Pregnancy and Preterm Birth in Women Referred to

Health Centers of Ardabil. Iranian Red Crescent Medical Journal. 2015 Dec; 17(12)

35. Spiegler, E. Kim, Y. et al. Maternal-fetal transfer and metabolism of vitamin A and its precursor β-carotene in the developing tissues. Biochimica et Biophysica Acta (BBA) - Molecular and Cell Biology of Lipids. 2012 Jan; 1821(1): 88–98.

36. Hans, U. Edward, B. Regular vitamin C supplementation during pregnancy reduces hospitalization: outcomes of a Ugandan rural cohort study. The Pan African Medical Journal. May 2010.

37. Grigel, K. Pregnant Women Need More Protein. Study reports that current recommendations are inadequate. Natural Medicine Journal. August 2015 Vol. 7 Issue 8

38. Innis, S. Dietary omega 3 fatty acids and the developing brain. Brain Research. Volume 1237, 27 October 2008, Pages 35–43.

39. North Carolina State University. Compounds From Soy Affect Brain And Reproductive Development. Science Daily .Your source for the latest research news August 1, 2008

40. National Institute of Environmental Health Science. Soy Infant Formula. http://www.niehs.nih.gov/health/topics/agents/sya-soy-formula/

41. Park JH, Choi TS. Subcutaneous administration of monosodium glutamate to pregnant mice reduces weight gain in pups during lactation. Laboratory Animals. 2016 Apr;50(2):94-9

42. Bazer FW, Wu G, Johnson GA, Wang X. Environmental factors affecting pregnancy: endocrine disrupters, nutrients and metabolic pathways. Mol Cell Endocrinol. 2014 Dec;398(1-2):53-68

43. Sloboda DM, Li M, Patel R, Clayton ZE, Yap C, Vickers MH. Early life exposure to fructose and

offspring phenotype: implications for long term metabolic homeostasis. Journal of Obesity. 2014;2014:203474

44. Krajmalnik-Brown, R. et al. Gut bacteria in children with autism spectrum disorders: challenges and promise of studying how a complex community influences a complex disease. Microbial Ecology in Health and Disease. 2015; 26.

45. Zhang, Y, Li, S. et al. Impacts of Gut Bacteria on Human Health and Diseases. International Journal of Molecular Sciences. 2015 Apr; 16(4): 7493–7519.

46. Di Mascio D, Magro-Malosso ER. Et al. Exercise during pregnancy in normal-weight women and risk of preterm birth: a systematic review and meta-analysis of randomized controlled trials. American Journal Obstetrics and Gynecology. 2016 Jun 16.

47. Morris, M. et al. Folate and vitamin B-12 status in relation to anemia, macrocytosis, and cognitive impairment in older Americans in the age of folic acid fortification. The American Journal of Clinical Nutrition. January 2007
vol. 85 no. 1 193-200

48. Troen, A. Mitchell, B. et al. Unmetabolized Folic Acid in Plasma Is Associated with Reduced Natural Killer Cell Cytotoxicity among Postmenopausal Women. The Journal of Nutrition. January 2006 vol. 136 no. 1 189-194

49. Hirsch S, Sanchez H, Albala C, de la Maza MP, Barrera G, Leiva L, Bunout D. Colon cancer in Chile before and after the start of the flour fortification program with folic acid. European Journal Gastroenterology Hepatology. 2009 Apr;21(4):436-9

50. Figueiredo, J. et al. Folic Acid and Risk of Prostate Cancer: Results From a Randomized Clinical Trial. Journal of the National Cancer Institute. (2009) 101 (6): 432-435.

51. Vitamin D council. Vitamin D during pregnancy and breastfeeding. January 30, 2013. http://www.vitamindcouncil.org/further-topics/vitamin-d-during-pregnancy-and-breastfeeding/

52. Wagner CL, Hulsey TC, Fanning D, Ebeling M, Hollis BW. High-dose vitamin D3 supplementation in a cohort of breastfeeding mothers and their infants: a 6-month follow-up pilot study. Breastfeeding Medicine. 2006 Summer;1(2):59-70.

53. Moushumi, L., et. al. Assessment of Vitamin D status In Patients of Chronic Low Back Pain of Unknown Etiology. Indian Journal of Clinical Biochemistry, 2015

54. Hunter, K. Probiotics in the first trimester for post pregnancy weight loss? Australian Journal of Medical Herbalism. Jun 22, 2009

55. Reed, R. Johnson-Cash, J. The Human Microbiome: considerations for pregnancy, birth and early mothering. MidwifeThinking. January 15, 2014

56. Almonte RA, Heath DL, Whitehall J, Russell MJ, Patole S, Vink R. Gestational magnesium deficiency is deleterious to fetal outcome. Biology of the Neonate. 1999 Jul;76(1):26-32

57. Bullarbo M, Ödman N, Nestler A. et al. Magnesium supplementation to prevent high blood pressure in pregnancy: a randomised placebo control trial. Archives of Gynecology Obstetrics. 2013 Dec;288(6):1269-74

58. Drews K. Folate metabolism--epigenetic role of choline and vitamin B12 during pregnancy. Ginekol Pol. 2015 Dec;86(12):940-6.

59. Leung,A, Pearce, E. Braverman, L. Iodine Nutrition in Pregnancy and Lactation. Endocrinol Metab Clin North Am. 2011 Dec; 40(4): 765–777.

60. Monahan, M. et al. Costs and benefits of iodine supplementation for pregnant women in a mildly to moderately iodine-deficient population: a modelling

analysis. The Lancet Diabetes & Endocrinology. Volume 3, No. 9, p715–722, September 2015.

61. Liew, Z. Ritz, B . Virk, J. Olsen J. Maternal use of acetaminophen during pregnancy and risk of autism spectrum disorders in childhood: A Danish national birth cohort study. Autism Research. 2015 Dec 21.

62. Brandlistuen, R. et al. Prenatal paracetamol exposure and child neurodevelopment: a sibling-controlled cohort study. International Journal of Epidemiology 2013;42:1702–1713.

63. Stergiakouli, E. et al. Association of Acetaminophen Use During Pregnancy With Behavioral Problems in Childhood. JAMA Pediatrics. August 15, 2016.

64. Liew, Z., Ritz, B. Et at. Acetaminophen Use During Pregnancy, Behavioral Problems, and Hyperkinetic Disorders. JAMA Pediatrics. 2014;168(4):313-320.

65. Center for Disease Control and Prevention. Questions and Answers About Vaccines During Pregnancy. http://www.cdc.gov/vaccinesafety/concerns/vaccines-during-pregnancy.html

66. Miller, N. Goldman, G. Infant mortality rates regressed against number of vaccine doses routinely given: Is there a biochemical or synergistic toxicity? Human Experimental Toxicology. 2011 Sep; 30(9): 1420–1428.

67. Central Intelligence Agency. Infant Mortality Rate. 2015. https://www.cia.gov/library/publications/the-world-factbook/rankorder/2091rank.html

68. Frohlich, T. Kent, A, Allen, A. Countries Spending the Most on Health Care. July 7, 2014. 24/7 Wall St. http://247wallst.com/special-report/2014/07/07/countries-spending-the-most-on-health-care/5/

69. News Medical. Life Sciences and Medicine. Stress during pregnancy affects babies' brain development.

June 23, 2015. http://www.news-medical.net/news/20150623/Stress-during-pregnancy-affects-babies-brain-development.aspx

70. Gitau R, Fisk NM, Teixeira JM, Cameron A, Glover V. Fetal hypothalamic-pituitary-adrenal stress responses to invasive procedures are independent of maternal responses. Journal Clinical Endocrinology and Metabolism. 2001 Jan;86(1):104-9

71. Sandman CA, Glynn L, Schetter CD, Wadhwa P, Garite T, Chicz-DeMet A, Hobel C. Elevated maternal cortisol early in pregnancy predicts third trimester levels of placental corticotropin releasing hormone (CRH): priming the placental clock. Peptides. 2006 Jun;27(6):1457-63

72. Buss, C. Davis, E. Et al. High pregnancy anxiety during mid-gestation is associated with decreased gray matter density in 6-9 year-old children. Psychoneuroendocrinology. 2010 Jan; 35(1): 141–153.

73. Kane, H. Schetter, C, Glynn, L. Et al. Pregnancy Anxiety and Prenatal Cortisol Trajectories. Biol Psychol. 2014 Jul; 100: 13–19.

74. Newsweek. How Stress Can Affect You and Your Unborn Baby. 3/22/15 http://www.newsweek.com/how-calm-your-anxiety-during-pregnancy-315242

75. Doyle, C. Werner, E. Et al. Pregnancy Distress Gets Under Fetal Skin: Maternal Ambulatory Assessment & Sex Differences in Prenatal Development. Dev Psychobiol. 2015 Jul; 57(5): 607–625.

76. Allister L, Lester BM, Carr S, Liu J. The effects of maternal depression on fetal heart rate response to vibroacoustic stimulation. Dev Neuropsychol. 2001;20(3):639-51.

77. Glover, V. The Effects of Maternal Anxiety or Stress during Pregnancy on the Fetus and the Long-Term

Development of the Child. Nutrition and Health July 2007 vol. 19 no. 1-2 61-62

78. Li, Y. Gonzalez, P. Zhang,L. Fetal Stress and Programming of Hypoxic/Ischemic-Sensitive Phenotype in the Neonatal Brain: Mechanisms and Possible Interventions. Prog Neurobiol. 2012 Aug; 98(2): 145–165.

79. Exercise during pregnancy and the postpartum period. ACOG Technical Bulletin Number 189-- February 1994. Int J Gynaecol Obstet. 1994 Apr;45(1):65-70

80. Mayo Clinic. Miscarriage. http://www.mayoclinic.org/diseases-conditions/pregnancy-loss-miscarriage/home/ovc-20213664

81. Tomic, V. Sporis, G. Et al. The effect of maternal exercise during pregnancy on abnormal fetal growth. Croatian Medical Journal. 2013 Aug; 54(4): 362–368.

82. Thorell E, Goldsmith L, Weiss G, Kristiansson P. Physical fitness, serum relaxin and duration of gestation. BMC Pregnancy Childbirth. 2015 Aug 14;15:168

83. Wang TW, Apgar BS. Exercise during pregnancy. American Family Physician. 1998 Apr 15;57(8):1846-52

84. Milunsky A, Ulcickas M, Rothman KJ, Willett W, Jick SS, Jick H. Maternal heat exposure and neural tube defects. JAMA. 1992 Aug 19;268(7):882-5

85. Bung P, Artal R, Khodiguian N, Kjos S. Exercise in gestational diabetes. An optional therapeutic approach? Diabetes. 1991 Dec;40 Suppl 2:182-5

86. Clapp JF 3rd, Little KD. Effect of recreational exercise on pregnancy weight gain and subcutaneous fat deposition. Medicine and Science in Sports Exercise. 1995 Feb;27(2):170-7

87. Wolfe LA, Brenner IK, Mottola MF. Maternal exercise, fetal well-being and pregnancy outcome. Exercise Sport Science Reviews. 1994;22:145-94.
88. Marcoux S, Brisson J, Fabia J. The effect of leisure time physical activity on the risk of pre-eclampsia and gestational hypertension. Journal of Epidemiology and Community Health. 1989 Jun;43(2):147-52.
89. American Pregnancy Association. Effects of Exercise on Pregnancy. http://americanpregnancy.org/pregnancy-health/effects-of-exercise-on-pregnancy/
90. Hammer, R. Perkins, J. Parr, R. Exercise During the Childbearing Year. Journal of Perinatal Education. 2000 Winter; 9(1): 1–14
91. American College of Obstetricians and Gynecologists. Exercise After Pregnancy. June 2015. http://www.acog.org/Patients/FAQs/Exercise-After-Pregnancy
92. Davis K, Goodman SH, Leiferman J, Taylor M, Dimidjian S. A randomized controlled trial of yoga for pregnant women with symptoms of depression and anxiety. Complementary Therapies in Clinical Practice. 2015 Aug;21(3):166-72.
93. Cammu H, Van Nylen M. Pelvic floor muscle exercises: 5 years later. Urology. 1995 Jan;45(1):113-7
94. Spinning Babies. Pelvic Tilt. http://spinningbabies.com/learn-more/techniques/other-techniques/pelvic-tilt/
95. Dimidjian S, Goodman SH, Felder JN, Gallop R, Brown AP, Beck A. Staying well during pregnancy and the postpartum: A pilot randomized trial of mindfulness-based cognitive therapy for the prevention of depressive relapse/recurrence. Journal of Consulting and Clinical Psychology. 2016 Feb;84(2):134-45

96. Marc I, Toureche N, Ernst E, Hodnett ED, Blanchet C, Dodin S, Njoya MM. Mind-body interventions during pregnancy for preventing or treating women's anxiety. Cochrane Database Systematic Reviews. 2011 Jul 6;(7):

97. Tiralongo E. Wee SS., Lea RA. Elderberry Supplementation Reduces Cold Duration and Symptoms in Air-Travellers: A Randomized, Double-Blind Placebo-Controlled Clinical Trial. Nutrients. 2016 Mar 24;8(4):182.

98. Giles JT, Palat CT 3rd, Chien SH, Chang ZG, Kennedy DT. Evaluation of echinacea for treatment of the common cold. Pharmacotherapy. 2000 Jun;20(6):690-7.

99. Block KI, Mead MN. Immune system effects of echinacea, ginseng, and astragalus: a review. Integrative Cancer Therapies. 2003 Sep;2(3):247-67

100. Carr AB, Einstein R, Lai LY, Martin NG, Starmer GA. Vitamin C and the common cold: using identical twins as controls. Medical Journal Australia. 1981 Oct 17;2(8):411-2

101. Hemilä H, Petrus EJ, Fitzgerald JT, Prasad A. Zinc acetate lozenges for treating the common cold: an individual patient data meta-analysis. British Journal of Clinical Pharmacology. 2016 July 5.

102. Lamberti LM, Fischer Walker CL, Black RE. Zinc Deficiency in Childhood and Pregnancy: Evidence for Intervention Effects and Program Responses. World Review Nutrition Diet. 2016;115:125-33.

103. Bode, A. Dong, Z. Herbal Medicine: Biomolecular and Clinical Aspects. 2nd edition. Benzie IFF, Wachtel-Galor S, editors. Boca Raton (FL): CRC Press/Taylor & Francis; 2011

104. University of Maryland Medical Center. Garlic. http://umm.edu/health/medical/altmed/herb/garlic

105. Harvard Health Publications; Harvard Medical School. How to boost your immune system. http://www.health.harvard.edu/staying-healthy/how-to-boost-your-immune-system

106. National Institutes of Health. Vitamin C. https://ods.od.nih.gov/factsheets/VitaminC-HealthProfessional/

107. Ko, S. Park, J. Et al. Antioxidant Effects of Spinach (Spinacia oleracea L.) Supplementation in Hyperlipidemic Rats. Preventive Nutrition and Food Science. 2014 Mar; 19(1): 19–26

108. Guggenheim, A. Wright, K. Zwickey, H. Immune Modulation From Five Major Mushrooms: Application to Integrative Oncology. Integrative Medicine: A Clinician's Journal (Encinitas). 2014 Feb; 13(1): 32–44

109. MedlinePlus. NIH: US National Library of Medicine. Exercise and immunity. https://www.nlm.nih.gov/medlineplus/ency/article/007165.htm

110. Stanford Medicine. Immune systems of healthy adults 'remember' germs to which they've never been exposed, Stanford study finds. https://med.stanford.edu/news/all-news/2013/02/immune-systems-of-healthy-adults-remember-germs-to-which-theyve-never-been-exposed-stanford-study-finds.html

111. Vitamin D Council. GERD and heartburn: Medication reduces magnesium stores. https://www.vitamindcouncil.org/blog/gerd-and-heartburn-medication-reduces-magnesium-stores/

112. Gandhi NY, Sharif WK, Chadha S, Shakher J. A patient on long-term proton pump inhibitors develops sudden seizures and encephalopathy: an unusual presentation of hypomagnesaemia. Case Rep Gastrointest Med. 2012;2012:632721

113. Lisi AJ. Chiropractic spinal manipulation for low back pain of pregnancy: a retrospective case series. Journal of Midwifery and Women's Health. 2006 Jan-Feb;51(1):e7-10.

114. Goertz, C. Long, C. Et al. Adding Chiropractic Manipulative Therapy to Standard Medical Care for Patients With Acute Low Back Pain: Results of a Pragmatic Randomized Comparative Effectiveness Study. Spine. 15 April 2013 - Volume 38 - Issue 8 - p 627–634.

115. Sadr, S. Pourkiani-Allah-Abad, N, Stuber, K. The treatment experience of patients with low back pain during pregnancy and their chiropractors: a qualitative study. Chiropractic & Manual Therapies201220:32

116. American Pregnancy Association. Massage and Pregnancy – Prenatal Massage. http://americanpregnancy.org/pregnancy-health/prenatal-massage/

117. Kragstrupt, T. Vitamin D supplementation for patients with chronic pain. Scandinavian Journal Primary Health Care. 2011 Mar; 29(1): 4–5.

118. Lodh M, Goswami B, Mahajan RD, Sen D, Jajodia N, Roy A. Assessment of Vitamin D status In Patients of Chronic Low Back Pain of Unknown Etiology. Indian Journal Clinical Biochemistry. 2015 Apr;30(2):174-9.

119. Vitamin D Council. Vitamin D during pregnancy and breastfeeding. http://www.vitamindcouncil.org/further-topics/vitamin-d-during-pregnancy-and-breastfeeding/

120. Tilbrook, H, Et al. Yoga for Chronic Low Back Pain: A Randomized Trial. Annals of Internal Medicine. 1 November 2011, Vol 155, No. 9.

121. Alcantara, J. Cossette, M. Intractable migraine headaches during pregnancy under chiropractic care. Complementary Therapies in Clinical Practice. Volume 15, Issue 4, November 2009, Pages 192–197

122. American Pregnancy Association. Fatigue During Pregnancy. http://americanpregnancy.org/your-pregnancy/fatigue-during-pregnancy/

123. Underactive Thyroid: Overview. PubMedHealth. U.S. National Library of Medicine. October 8, 2014.

124. American Pregnancy Association. Pregnancy and Hair Loss. http://americanpregnancy.org/pregnancy-health/hair-loss-during-pregnancy/

125. ACOG. Depression During Pregnancy: Treatment Recommendations. August 21, 2009

126. Glynn, L. How Pregnancy Changes a Woman's Brain. Association for Psychological Science. December 20, 2011

127. American Pregnancy Association. Spotting During Pregnancy. http://americanpregnancy.org/pregnancy-concerns/spotting-during-pregnancy/

128. Cochrane Database of Systematic Reviews. Magnesium for muscle cramps. Oct. 11, 2011.

129. American Pregnancy Association. Treating Varicose Veins Naturally During Pregnancy. http://americanpregnancy.org/naturally/treating-varicose-veins-naturally-during-pregnancy/

130. Renault KM, Carlsen EM, Nørgaard K. Et al. Intake of Sweets, Snacks and Soft Drinks Predicts Weight Gain in Obese Pregnant Women: Detailed Analysis of the Results of a Randomised Controlled Trial. PLoS One. 2015 Jul 20;10(7)

131. Farland LV, Rifas-Shiman SL, Gillman MW. Early Pregnancy Cravings, Dietary Intake, and Development of Abnormal Glucose Tolerance. Journal of the Academy of Nutrition Diet. 2015 Dec;115(12):1958-1964

132. Abumaria N, Yin B, Zhang L, Et al. Effects of elevation of brain magnesium on fear conditioning, fear extinction, and synaptic plasticity in the infralimbic prefrontal cortex and lateral amygdala.

Journal of Neuroscience. 2011 Oct 19;31(42):14871-81

133. Harvard Health Publications. Chromium supplements: chromium, diabetes, and weight loss. http://www.health.harvard.edu/press_releases/chromium-supplements

134. Plants in Action. Carbon accumulation. 11.4.1. http://plantsinaction.science.uq.edu.au/edition1/?q=content/11-4-1-carbon-accumulation

135. Institute of Medicine (US) Committee on Nutritional Status During Pregnancy and Lactation. Nutrition During Pregnancy: Part I Weight Gain: Part II Nutrient Supplements. Washington (DC): National Academies Press (US); 1990

136. Mayo Clinic. Sodium: How to tame your salt habit. Find out how much sodium you really need, what high-sodium foods to avoid, and ways to prepare and serve foods without adding sodium. Nutrition and healthy eating. April 16, 2016. http://www.mayoclinic.org/healthy-lifestyle/nutrition-and-healthy-eating/in-depth/sodium/art-20045479

137. Orloff, N, Hormes, J. Pickles and ice cream! Food cravings in pregnancy: hypotheses, preliminary evidence, and directions for future research. Frontiers in Psychology. 2014; 5: 1076

138. Khamis MA, Mustafa MF, Mohamed SN, Toson MM. Influence of gestational period on sexual behavior. Journal of Egypt Public Health Assoc. 2007;82(1-2):65-90

139. Mårdh PA, Colleen S. Antimicrobial activity of human seminal fluid. Scandinavian Journal Urology and Nephrology. 1975;9(1):17-23.

140. Chantler PD, Melenovsky V. Et al. The sex-specific impact of systolic hypertension and systolic blood pressure on arterial-ventricular coupling at rest and

during exercise. American Journal Physiology. Heart Circulatory Physiology. 2008 Jul;295(1):H145-53
141. Benefits of love and sex. NHS Choices. http://www.nhs.uk/Livewell/Goodsex/Pages/Valentine sDay.aspx
142. Sex hormones and the immune response in humans. Human Reproduction Update. Volume 11, Issue 4. Pp. 411-423.
143. Charnetski, C. Brennan, F. Sexual Frequency and Salivary Immunoglobulin A (IgA). Psychology Reports. June 2004 vol. 94 no. 3 839-844
144. Koelman CA, Coumans AB. Et al. Correlation between oral sex and a low incidence of preeclampsia: a role for soluble HLA in seminal fluid? Journal of Reproductive Immunology. 2000 Mar;46(2):155-66.
145. Whipple, B. Komisaruk, B. Elevation of Pain Threshold by Vaginal Stimulation in Women. Pain. May 1985.
146. Leeners, B et al. The Quality of Sexual Experience in Women Correlates with Post-Orgasmic Prolactin Surges: Results from an Experimental Prototype Study. The Journal of Sexual Medicine. Volume 10, Issue. May 2013 .Pages 1313–1319
147. Kavanagh J, Kelly AJ, Thomas J. Sexual intercourse for cervical ripening and induction of labour. Cochrane Database Syst Rev. 2001
148. Golmakani, N. et al. The effect of pelvic floor muscle exercises program on sexual self-efficacy in primiparous women after delivery. Iran Journal of Nursing and Midwifery Research. 2015 May-Jun; 20(3): 347–353.
149. Read, J. Klebanoff, M. Sexual intercourse during pregnancy and preterm delivery: Effects of vaginal microorganisms. American Journal of Obstetrics and

Gynecology. February 1993Volume 168, Issue 2, Pages 514–519

150. Brown, B. Sexual Intercourse and Orgasm During Late Pregnancy May Have a Protective Effect Against Preterm Delivery. Guttmacher Institute. Volume 33, Issue 4 .July/August 2001   Pages 180 - 181

151. Behrman RE, Butler AS. Behavioral and Psychosocial Contributors to Preterm Birth. Institute of Medicine (US) Committee on Understanding Premature Birth and Assuring Healthy Outcomes. Washington (DC): National Academies Press (US); 2007

152. Sayle AE, Savitz DA. Et al. Sexual activity during late pregnancy and risk of preterm delivery. Obstetrics and Gynecology. 2001 Feb;97(2):283-9.

153. Planned Parenthood. The Health Benefits of Sexual Expression. Published in Cooperation with the Society for the Scientific Study of Sexuality. July 2007. https://www.plannedparenthood.org/files/3413/9611/7801/Benefits_Sex_07_07.pdf

154. Environmental Working Group. Body Burden:The Pollution in Newborns. A benchmark investigation of industrial chemicals, pollutants and pesticides in umbilical cord blood. http://www.ewg.org/research/body-burden-pollution-newborns

155. Geirsson RT. Intrauterine volume in pregnancy. Acta Obstetricia Gynecologica Scandinavica Supplement 1986;136:1-74.

156. University of California San Francisco Medical Center. Conception: How It Works. https://www.ucsfhealth.org/education/conception_how_it_works/

157. Mimeault, M. Batra, S. GREAT PROMISE OF TISSUE-RESIDENT ADULT STEM/PROGENITOR

CELLS IN TRANSPLANTATION AND CANCER THERAPIES. Adv Exp Med Biol. 2012; 741: 171–186.

158. Rochman, B. Can Mail-In Menstrual Blood Banks Help Save Lives? Time Magazine. March 9th, 2011. http://healthland.time.com/2011/03/09/stem-cells-from-menstrual-blood-strange-but-true/

159. Balan, S. Use of Menstrual Blood to Cure Diseases - Medicine Therapy Applications. Biotech Articles. Nov. 9, 2011, http://www.biotecharticles.com/Healthcare-Article/Use-of-Menstrual-Blood-to-Cure-Diseases-Medicine-Therapy-Applications-1033.html

160. Kumar, P. Magon, N. Hormones in pregnancy. Nigerian Medical Journal. 2012 Oct-Dec; 53(4): 179–183.

161. Barbagallo, M. et al. Vascular Effects of Progesterone. Role of Cellular Calcium Regulation. American Heart Association. Hypertension. 2001; 37: 142-147.

162. Breeze, C. Early pregnancy bleeding. Australian Family Physician. 2016 May;45(5):283-6.

163. Sanghavi, M. Rutherford, J. Cardiovascular Physiology of Pregnancy. Circulation. September 16, 2014, Volume 130, Issue 12

164. US Department of Health and Human Services | National Institutes of Health. Recent NICHD Research Reveals that Gaining More Than the Recommended Weight During Pregnancy Increases the Risk for Complications. https://www.nichd.nih.gov/news/resources/spotlight/Pages/082813-pregnancy-weight.aspx

165. Jašarević, E. Howerton, C. Et al. Alterations in the Vaginal Microbiome by Maternal Stress Are Associated With Metabolic Reprogramming of the

Offspring Gut and Brain. Endocrine Society. May 15, 2015

166. U.S. National Library of Medicine. Fetal development.
https://medlineplus.gov/ency/article/002398.htm

167. National Health Service of England. What is the amniotic sac?
http://www.nhs.uk/NHSEngland/AboutNHSservices/Pages/NHSServices.aspx

168. Jaddoe, V. Et al. First trimester fetal growth restriction and cardiovascular risk factors in school age children: population based cohort study. BMJ 2014; 348.

169. Kalb, C. Fetal Armor. Scientific American 306, 72 - 73 (2012).
http://www.nature.com/scientificamerican/journal/v306/n2/full/scientificamerican0212-72.html

170. Mor, G. Cardenas, I. The Immune System in Pregnancy: A Unique Complexity. American Journal Reproductive Immunology. 2010 Jun; 63(6): 425–433.

171. Dawe, G. Tan, X. Xiao, Z. Cell Migration from Baby to Mother. Cell Adhesion and Migration. 2007 Jan-Mar; 1(1): 19–27.

172. Walker CK, Krakowiak P, Baker A. Preeclampsia, placental insufficiency, and autism spectrum disorder or developmental delay. JAMA Pediatrics. 2015 Feb;169(2):154-62

173. Wang Y, Zhao S. Chapter 2 Placental Blood Circulation. Vascular Biology of the Placenta. San Rafael (CA): Morgan & Claypool Life Sciences; 2010.

174. US Department of Health and Human Services. National Institutes of Health. The Human Placenta Project.
https://www.nichd.nih.gov/research/HPP/Pages/default.aspx

175. Mayo Clinic. Fetal development: The 2nd trimester. Fetal development takes on new meaning in the second trimester. Highlights might include finding out your baby's sex and feeling your baby move. http://www.mayoclinic.org/healthy-lifestyle/pregnancy-week-by-week/in-depth/fetal-development/art-20046151

176. American Pregnancy Association. Fetal Development: Second Trimester. http://americanpregnancy.org/while-pregnant/second-trimester/

177. Burd, I. Finke, A. University of Rochester Medical Center. The Second Trimester. Prenatal visits during the second trimester. https://www.urmc.rochester.edu/encyclopedia/content.aspx?contenttypeid=85&contentid=P01234

178. American Pregnancy Association. Gestational Diabetes. http://americanpregnancy.org/pregnancy-complications/gestational-diabetes/

179. The HAPO Study Cooperative Research Group. Hyperglycemia and Adverse Pregnancy Outcomes. New England Journal of Medicine. 2008; 358:1991-2002. May 8, 2008

180. Aparicio NJ, Joao MA, Cortelezzi M. Pregnant women with impaired tolerance to an oral glucose load in the afternoon: evidence suggesting that they behave metabolically as patients with gestational diabetes. American Journal of Obstetrics and Gynecology. 1998 May;178(5):1059-66.

181. American Pregnancy Association. Glucose Tolerance Test. http://americanpregnancy.org/prenatal-testing/glucose-tolerence-test/

182. American Diabetes Association. How to Treat Gestational Diabetes.

http://www.diabetes.org/diabetes-basics/gestational/how-to-treat-gestational.html

183. Wilcox, G. Insulin and Insulin Resistance. Clinical Biochemistry Reviews. 2005 May; 26(2): 19–39.

184. Sahariah, SA, Potdar, RD. Et al. A Daily Snack Containing Leafy Green Vegetables, Fruit, and Milk before and during Pregnancy Prevents Gestational Diabetes in a Randomized, Controlled Trial in Mumbai, India. The Journal of Nutrition. 2016 Jul;146(7):1453S-60S

185. Bodnar, L. Platt, R. Simham, H. Early-Pregnancy Vitamin D Deficiency and Risk of Preterm Birth Subtypes. Obstetrics & Gynecology: February 2015 - Volume 125 - Issue 2 - p 439–447

186. Zhang, C, Williams, MA. Maternal plasma ascorbic Acid (vitamin C) and risk of gestational diabetes mellitus. Epidemiology. 2004 Sep;15(5):597-604.

187. Coustan, D. Can a Dietary Supplement Prevent Gestational Diabetes Mellitus? Diabetes Care. 2013 Apr; 36(4): 777–779.

188. Liang, HY, Hou, F. Clinical evaluation of the antioxidant activity of astragalus in women with gestational diabetes. Nan Fang Yi Ke Da Xue Xue Bao. 2009 Jul;29(7):1402-4.

189. Newhham, JP. Evans, S. et all. Effects of frequent ultrasound during pregnancy: a randomised controlled trial. The Lancet. Volume 342, Issue 8876, 9 October 1993, Pages 887-891

190. Ang, E. Gluncic, V. et al. Prenatal exposure to ultrasound waves impacts neuronal migration in mice. Proceedings of the National Academy of Sciences of the United States of America. August 22, 2006. vol. 103 no. 34

191. Mayo Clinic. Tests and Procedures. Ultrasound. http://www.mayoclinic.org/tests-procedures/ultrasound/basics/definition/prc-20020341

192. Butt, K. Lin, K. Determination of Gestational Age by Ultrasound. J Obstet Gynaecol Can 2014;36(2):171–181

193. NHS choices. Your health, your choices. The pregnancy dating scan. 02/25/2015 http://www.nhs.uk/Conditions/pregnancy-and-baby/Pages/dating-scan-ultrasound-10-11-12-13-weeks-pregnant.aspx

194. Advanced Women's Imaging. http://www.advancedwomensimaging.com.au/first-trimester-dating-ultrasound

195. The International Society of Ultrasound in Obstetrics and Gynecology (ISUOG) Practice Guidelines: performance of first-trimester fetal ultrasound scan. Ultrasound Obstet Gynecol 2013; 41: 102–113

196. NHS Choices. Your health, your choice. Pregnancy and baby. 02/09/2015 http://www.nhs.uk/Conditions/pregnancy-and-baby/pages/screening-amniocentesis-downs-syndrome.aspx#close

197. Bricker, L. et al. Ultrasound screening in pregnancy: a systematic review of the clinical effectiveness,cost-effectiveness and women's views. Health Technology Assessment 2000; Vol.4: No.16

198. Pahuja, M. 18-20 Week Screening Pregnancy Ultrasound. Inside Radiology. The Royal Australian and New Zealand College of Radiologists. http://www.insideradiology.com.au/pages/view.php?T id=68#.V-FVHTgtapp

199. American Pregnancy Association. Biophysical Profile. http://americanpregnancy.org/prenatal-testing/biophysical-profile/

200. American Pregnancy Association. Fetal Non-Stress Test (NST). http://americanpregnancy.org/prenatal-testing/non-stress-test/

201. Johns Hopkins Medicine. Pregnancy: The Third Trimester.
http://www.hopkinsmedicine.org/healthlibrary/conditions/pregnancy_and_childbirth/the_third_trimester_85,p01242/

202. Knudsen A. Lebech M. Hansen M. Upper gastrointestinal symptoms in the third trimester of the normal pregnancy. European Journal Obstetrics Gynecology Reproductive Biology. 1995 May;60(1):29-33

203. Khazaie H. Ghadami MR. et al. Insomnia treatment in the third trimester of pregnancy reduces postpartum depression symptoms: a randomized clinical trial. Psychiatry Research. 2013 Dec 30;210(3):901-5.

204. National Institutes of Health. U.S. National Library of Medicine.   Fetal development.
https://medlineplus.gov/ency/article/002398.htm

205. American Pregnancy Association. Fetal Development: Third Trimester.
http://americanpregnancy.org/while-pregnant/third-trimester/

206. Johns Hopkins Medicine. Pregnancy: The Third Trimester.
http://www.hopkinsmedicine.org/healthlibrary/conditions/pregnancy_and_childbirth/the_third_trimester_85,P01242/

207. Mayo Clinic. Pregnancy week by week. July, 11. 2014 http://www.mayoclinic.org/healthy-lifestyle/pregnancy-week-by-week/in-depth/fetal-development/art-20045997?pg=2

208. Leonhardt, D. Cox, A. Heavier Babies do Better in School. New York Times. 10/10/2014.
http://www.nytimes.com/2014/10/12/upshot/heavier-babies-do-better-in-school.html?_r=1

209. International Chiropractic Pediatric Association. The Webster Technique: A Chiropractic Technique. J Manipulative Physiol Ther. 2002 Jul-Aug;25(6): E1-9

210. Center for Disease Control and Prevention. Group B Strep (GBS). http://www.cdc.gov/groupbstrep/about/infection.html

211. Young BC. Dodge LE. Et al. Evaluation of a rapid, real-time intrapartum group B streptococcus assay. American Journal Obstetrics Gynecology. 2011 Oct;205(4):372.e1-6

212. Darling, E. Saurette, K. Group B Streptococcus: Prevention and Management in Labour. Association of Ontario Midwives. Jan. 2010

213. National Institutes of Health. U.S. National Library of Medicine. Group B streptococcal septicemia of the newborn. https://medlineplus.gov/ency/article/001366.htm

214. Adair CE. Kowalsky L. et al. Risk factors for early-onset group B streptococcal disease in neonates: a population-based case-control study. Canadian Medical Association Journal. 2003 Aug 5;169(3):198-203.

215. Dinsmoor MJ. Viloria R. Lief L. Elder S. Use of intrapartum antibiotics and the incidence of postnatal maternal and neonatal yeast infections. Obstetrics and Gynecology. 2005 Jul;106(1):19-22

216. PubMed Health. US National Library of Medicine. Pregnancy and Birth: Epidurals and painkillers for labor pain. July 19, 2012. http://www.ncbi.nlm.nih.gov/pubmedhealth/PMH0072751/

217. Sears, W. 7 Common Types of Epidural Births. 2016 http://www.askdrsears.com/topics/pregnancy-childbirth/pregnancy-concerns/managing-pain-during-childbirth/7-common-types

218. Drugs.com. Novocain.
https://www.drugs.com/pro/novocain.html

219. Alfirevic Z. Kelly AJ. Dowswell T. Intravenous oxytocin alone for cervical ripening and induction of labour. Cochrane Database Syst Rev. 2009 Oct 7

220. Gimovsky, AC. Guarente, J. Berghella, V. Prolonged second stage in nulliparous with epidurals: a systematic review. Journal of Maternal- Fetal and Neonatal Medicine. 2016 May 5:1-5

221. American Pregnancy Association. Epidural Anesthesia. 2016.
http://americanpregnancy.org/labor-and-birth/epidural/

222. Greenwell, E. et al. Intrapartum Temperature Elevation, Epidural Use, and Adverse Outcome in Term Infants. PEDIATRICS 129(2):e447-54 · February 2012

223. Torvaldsen, S. et al. Intrapartum epidural analgesia and breastfeeding: a prospective cohort study. International Breastfeeding Journal. Dec. 11, 2006

224. Dozier, A. et al. Labor Epidural Anesthesia, Obstetric Factors and Breastfeeding Cessation. Maternal and Child Health Journal. 2013 May; 17(4): 689–698.

225. Tsuzuki, Y. Yamashita, Y. Pain-reducing anesthesia prevents oxidative stress in human term placenta. Journal Clinical Biochemical Nutrition. 2016 Mar;58(2):156-60

226. Center for Disease Control and Prevention. Births - Method of Delivery. July 6, 2016.
http://www.cdc.gov/nchs/fastats/delivery.htm

227. Kassebaum, N. et al. Global, regional, and national levels and causes of maternal mortality during 1990–2013: a systematic analysis for the Global Burden of Disease Study 2013. The Lancet. Volume 384, No. 9947, p980–1004, 13 September 2014.

228. World Health Organization.
http://www.who.int/gho/maternal_health/countries/usa
.pdf?ua=1

229. Family Centered Cesarean. What is Family
Centered Cesarean? February 8, 2015
https://familycenteredcesarean.com/2015/02/08/what-
is-family-centered-cesarean/

230. Smith J, Plaat F, Fisk N. The natural caesarean: a
woman-centred technique. BJOG 2008;115:1037–
1042.

231. Neu, J. Rushing, J. Cesarean versus Vaginal
Delivery: Long term infant outcomes and the Hygiene
Hypothesis. Clin Perinatol. 2011 Jun; 38(2): 321–
331.

232. Molloy, A. Mothers facing C-sections look to vaginal
'seeding' to boost their babies' health. The Guardian.
Aug. 17, 2015

233. Hung, KJ. Berg, O. Early skin-to-skin after cesarean
to improve breastfeeding. MCN American Journal
Maternal Child Nursing. 2011 Sep-Oct;36(5):318-24

234. Stevens, J. Schmied, V. Burns, E. Dahlen, H.
Immediate or early skin-to-skin contact after a
Caesarean section: a review of the literature. Matern
Child Nutr. 2014 Oct;10(4):456-73

235. Azad, M. et al. Gut microbiota of healthy Canadian
infants: profiles by mode of delivery and infant diet at
4 months. CMAJ March 19, 2013 vol. 185 no. 5

236. Penders, J. et al. Factors Influencing the
Composition of the Intestinal Microbiota in Early
Infancy. Pediatrics. August 2006, VOLUME 118 /
ISSUE 2

237. Prince, AL. Antony, KM. et al. The microbiome and
development: a mother's perspective. Semin Reprod
Med. 2014 Jan;32(1):14-22

238. De Weerth, C. et al. Intestinal Microbiota of Infants With Colic: Development and Specific Signatures. Pediatrics. January 2013

239. Rettner, R. Colicky Babies May Have Wrong Bacteria. Live Science. January 16, 2013. http://www.livescience.com/26312-gut-bacteria-infant-colic.html

240. Tollin, M. et al. Vernix caseosa as a multi-component defence system based on polypeptides, lipids, and their interactions. Cellular and Molecular Life Sciences. 2005 Oct; 62(19-20): 2390–2399.

241. Ajslev,TA. Andersen, CS. Et al. Childhood overweight after establishment of the gut microbiota: the role of delivery mode, pre-pregnancy weight and early administration of antibiotics. International Journal of Obesity (2011) 35, 522–529

242. Gregory, S. Anthopolos, R. et al. Association of Autism With Induced or Augmented Childbirth in North Carolina Birth Record (1990-1998) and Education Research (1997-2007) Databases. JAMA Pediatr. 2013;167(10):959-966

243. The American College of Obstetricians and Gynecologists. Ob-Gyns Redefine Meaning of "Term Pregnancy" Oct. 22, 2013. http://www.acog.org/About-ACOG/News-Room/News-Releases/2013/Ob-Gyns-Redefine-Meaning-of-Term-Pregnancy

244. Alfirevic, Z. Kelly, AJ. Dowswell, T. Intravenous oxytocin alone for cervical ripening and induction of labour. Cochrane Database Syst Rev. 2009 Oct 7.

245. Borggren, C. Pregnancy and chiropractic: a narrative review of the literature. Journal Chiropractic Medicine. 2007 Spring; 6(2): 70–74

246. Fallon, J. The effects of chiropractic treatment on pregnancy and labor: a comprehensive study.

Proceedings of the world chiropractic congress. 1991; 24-31

247. Lim, CE. Wilkinson, JM. Et al. Effect of acupuncture on induction of labor. Journal of Alternative Complement Med. 2009 Nov;15(11):1209-14

248. Al-Kuran, O. Al-Mehaisen, L. Et al. The effect of late pregnancy consumption of date fruit on labour and delivery. Journal of Obstetrics Gynecology. 2011;31(1):29-31

249. American Pregnancy Association. Rapid Labor. http://americanpregnancy.org/labor-and-birth/rapid-labor/

250. Suzuki, S. Clinical Significance of Precipitous Labor. Journal Clinical Medical Research. 2015 Mar; 7(3): 150–153.

251. Selander, J. et al. Human Maternal Placentophagy: A Survey of Self-Reported Motivations and Experiences Associated with Placenta Consumption. Ecology of Food and Nutrition Vol. 52 , Iss. 2,2013

252. Coyle, C. Hulse, K. et al. Placentophagy: therapeutic miracle or myth? Archives of Women's Mental Health. October 2015, Volume 18, Issue 5, pp 673–680

253. Perazzolo, S. Hirschmugl B. Et al. Computational modelling of fatty acid transport in the human placenta. Conf Proc IEEE Eng Med Biol Soc. 2015 Aug;2015:8054-7.

254. Young, SM. Gryder, LK. Presence and concentration of 17 hormones in human placenta processed for encapsulation and consumption. Placenta. 2016 Jul;43:86-9

255. Young, SM. Gryder, LK. Human placenta processed for encapsulation contains modest concentrations of 14 trace minerals and elements. Nutrition Research. 2016 Aug;36(8):872-8

256. Kristal, M. Thompson, A. Grishkat, H. Placenta ingestion enhances opiate analgesia in rats. Physiology & Behavior. Volume 35, Issue 4, October 1985, Pages 481–486

257. American Pregnancy Association. Baby Blues. http://americanpregnancy.org/first-year-of-life/baby-blues/

258. Brocklehurst, P. Hardy, P. et al. Perinatal and maternal outcomes by planned place of birth for healthy women with low risk pregnancies : the Birthplace in England national prospective cohort study. BMJ 2011; 343

259. Wiegers, TA, Keirse, M, et al. Outcome of planned home and planned hospital births in low risk pregnancies: prospective study in midwifery practices in the Netherlands. BMJ 1996; 313

260. Kay, BJ.Butter, IH. Women's health and social change: the case of lay midwives. International Journal Health Serv. 1988;18(2):223-36

261. Lewis, RM, McKoy, JN, Andrews JC, et al. Future Research Needs for Strategies To Reduce Cesarean Birth in Low-Risk Women: Identification of Future Research Needs From Comparative Effectiveness. Agency for Healthcare Research and Quality (US); 2012 Oct.

262. Sakala, C. Corry, M. Evidence-Based Maternity Care: What It Is and What It Can Achieve. Co-published by Childbirth Connection, the Reforming States Group, and the Milbank Memorial Fund. October 2008

263. Buckley, S. Epidurals: Risks and Concerns for Mother and Baby. Mothering No.133, Nov-Dec 2005, as "The Hidden Risks of Epidurals" and updated in Gentle Birth, Gentle Mothering: A Doctor's Guide to Natural Childbirth and Gentle Early Parenting Choices (Sarah J Buckley, Celestial Arts, 2009).

264. Gaskin, IM. Maternal Death in the United States: A Problem Solved or a Problem Ignored? Journal Perinatal Education. 2008 Spring; 17(2): 9–13.

265. Deneux-Tharaux, C. Carmona, E. Postpartum maternal mortality and cesarean delivery. Obstetrics and Gynecology. 2006 Sep;108(3 Pt 1):541-8

266. Davies, S. Troubled waters? AIMS Journal, 2011, Vol 23 No 4.

267. Unsworth, J. Vause, S. Meconium in labour. Obstetrics, Gynaecology & Reproductive Medicine. Volume 20, Issue 10, October 2010, Pages 289–294

268. Ghidini, A. Spong, C. Severe meconium aspiration syndrome is not caused by aspiration of meconium. American Journal Obstetrics, and Gynecology. October 2001Volume 185, Issue 4, Pages 931–938

269. Pintucci, A. Meregalli, V. Colombo, P. Fiorilli, A. Premature rupture of membranes at term in low risk women: how long should we wait in the "latent phase"? Journal Perinatal Medicine. 2014 Mar;42(2):189-96

270. Shalev, E. Peleg, D. et al. Comparison of 12- and 72-hour expectant management of premature rupture of membranes in term pregnancies. Obstet Gynecol. 1995 May;85(5 Pt 1):766-8.

271. Morales, WJ. Lazar, AJ. Expectant management of rupture of membranes at term. South Med J. 1986 Aug;79(8):955-8

272. Lenihan, JP Jr. Relationship of antepartum pelvic examinations to premature rupture of the membranes. Obstet Gynecol. 1984 Jan;63(1):33-7.

273. Hill, MJ. McWilliams, GD. The effect of membrane sweeping on prelabor rupture of membranes: a randomized controlled trial. Obstet Gynecol. 2008 Jun;111(6):1313-9

274. Moore, RM. Mansour, JM. Et al. The physiology of fetal membrane rupture: insight gained from the

determination of physical properties. Placenta. 2006 Nov-Dec;27(11-12):1037-51.

275. Pietrantoni, E. Et al. Docosahexaenoic Acid Supplementation during Pregnancy: A Potential Tool to Prevent Membrane Rupture and Preterm Labor. Int J Mol Sci. 2014 May; 15(5): 8024–8036.

276. Seaward, PG. Hannah, ME. Et al. International Multicentre Term Prelabor Rupture of Membranes Study: evaluation of predictors of clinical chorioamnionitis and postpartum fever in patients with prelabor rupture of membranes at term. American Journal Obstetrics Gynecology. 1997 Nov;177(5):1024-9.

277. Polin, R. Management of Neonates With Suspected or Proven Early-Onset Bacterial Sepsis. Pediatrics. May 2012, VOLUME 129 / ISSUE 5. From the American Academy of Pediatrics. Clinical Report

278. Rydhström, H. Ingemarsson, I. No benefit from conservative management in nulliparous women with premature rupture of the membranes (PROM) at term. A randomized study. Acta Obstet Gynecol Scand. 1991;70(7-8):543-7.

279. Caughey, A. Robinson, J. Norwitz, E. Contemporary Diagnosis and Management of Preterm Premature Rupture of Membranes. Rev Obstet Gynecol. 2008 Winter; 1(1): 11–22.

280. Mount Sinai Hospital. Preterm Premature Rupture Of Membranes (PPROM). http://www.mountsinai.org/patient-care/health-library/diseases-and-conditions/preterm-premature-rupture-of-membranes

281. Hadley, CB. Main, DM. Gabbe, SG. Risk Factors for preterm premature rupture of the fetal membranes. American Journal of Perinatology [1990, 7(4):374-379]

282. Ramsey, P. Nuthalapaty, F. et al. Contemporary management of preterm premature rupture of membranes (PPROM): A survey of maternal-fetal medicine providers. American Journal of Obstetrics and Gynecology. October 2004Volume 191, Issue 4, Pages 1497–1502
283. Catt, E. Chadha, R. et al. Management of Preterm Premature Rupture of Membranes: A Comparison of Inpatient and Outpatient Care. Journal Obstetrics Gynecology Canada. 2016 May;38(5):433-40
284. Ghomian, N. Hafizi, L. Takhti, Z. The Role of Vitamin C in Prevention of Preterm Premature Rupture of Membranes. Iran Red Crescent Med J. 2013 Feb; 15(2): 113–116.
285. March of Dimes. Preeclampsia. http://www.marchofdimes.org/complications/preeclampsia.aspx
286. Brantsaeter, A. Myhre, R. et al. Intake of Probiotic Food and Risk of Preeclampsia in Primiparous Women. The Norwegian Mother and Child Cohort Study. Am. J. Epidemiol. (2011) 174 (7): 807-815.
287. Qiu, C. Coughlin,KB. Et al. Dietary fiber intake in early pregnancy and risk of subsequent preeclampsia. Am J Hypertens. 2008 Aug;21(8):903-9
288. Frederick, IO. Williams, MA. Et al. Dietary fiber, potassium, magnesium and calcium in relation to the risk of preeclampsia. J Reprod Med. 2005 May;50(5):332-44.
289. Kisters, K. Barenbrock, M. Membrane, intracellular, and plasma magnesium and calcium concentrations in preeclampsia. Am J Hypertens (2000) 13 (7): 765-769.
290. 1.A. J. Webb, N. Patel, S. Loukogeorgakis, M. Okorie, Z. Aboud, S. Misra, R. Rashid, P. Miall, J. Deanfield, N. Benjamin, R. MacAllister, A. J. Hobbs, A. Ahluwalia. Acute Blood Pressure Lowering,

Vasoprotective, and Antiplatelet Properties of Dietary Nitrate via Bioconversion to Nitrite. Hypertension, 2008; 51 (3): 784

291. McCarty, M. Barruso-Aranda, J. Contreras, F. Spirulina for Prevention and Control of Preeclampsia. http://phycobilin.org/research/spirulina-PE.pdf.

292. Koelman, CA. Coumans, AB. Et Al. Correlation between oral sex and a low incidence of preeclampsia: a role for soluble HLA in seminal fluid? J Reprod Immunol. 2000 Mar;46(2):155-66.

293. Yeo, S. Davidge, S. et al. A comparison of walking versus stretching exercises to reduce the incidence of preeclampsia: a randomized clinical trial. Hypertens Pregnancy. 2008;27(2):113-30.

294. American Pregnancy Association. Prolonged Labor: Failure to Progress. http://americanpregnancy.org/labor-and-birth/prolonged-labor-failure-progress/

295. Frigo, MG. Larciprete, G. et al. Rebuilding the labor curve during neuraxial analgesia. J Obstet Gynaecol Res. 2011 Nov;37(11):1532-9

296. Hamilton, EF. Warrick, PA. et al. Assessing first-stage labor progression and its relationship to complications. Am J Obstet Gynecol. 2016 Mar;214(3):358

297. Mayo Clinic. Stages of labor and birth: Baby, it's time! Labor is a natural process. Here's what to expect during the three stages of labor and birth — and what you can do to promote comfort. http://www.mayoclinic.org/healthy-lifestyle/labor-and-delivery/in-depth/stages-of-labor/art-20046545?pg=1

298. National Institutes of Health. NIH Study Finds Women Spend Longer in Labor Now Than 50 Years Ago. March 30, 2012. https://www.nichd.nih.gov/news/releases/pages/0330 12-time-to-labor.aspx

299. Edgar, A. Anatomy of a Working Breast. NEW BEGINNINGS, Vol. 22 No. 2, March-April 2005, pp. 44-50

300. Hazzani, F. Is oronasopharyngeal suctioning necessary in neonatal resuscitation? J Clin Neonatol. 2013 Jul-Sep; 2(3): 118–120

301. Czarnecki, ML. Kaucic, CL. Infant nasal-pharyngeal suctioning: is it beneficial? Pediatr Nurs. 1999 Mar-Apr;25(2):193-6, 218

302. Healow, L. Hugh, R. Oral Aversion in the Breastfed Neonate. Breastfeeding Abstracts, August 2000, Volume 20, Number 1, pp. 3-4.

303. Waltman, PA. Brewer, JM. Building evidence for practice: a pilot study of newborn bulb suctioning at birth. J Midwifery Womens Health. 2004 Jan-Feb;49(1):32-8.

304. Neumann, I. Mounsey, A. Das, N. PURLs: Suctioning neonates at birth: Time to change our approach. J Fam Pract. 2014 Aug; 63(8): 461–462.

305. Said Habib, H.   Oxygen saturation trends in the first hour of life in healthy full-term neonates born at moderate altitude. Pak J Med Sci. 2013 Jul;29(4):903-6.

306. Murphy, P. The fetal circulation. Continuing Education Anesthesia Critical Care Pain (August 2005) 5 (4): 107-112.

307. Hutchon, D. Why do obstetricians and midwives still rush to clamp the cord? BMJ 2010; 341

308. Tolosa, JN. Park, DH. Et al. Mankind's first natural stem cell transplant. J Cell Mol Med. 2010 Mar;14(3):488-95

309. Mercer, JS. Erickson-Owens, DA. Rethinking placental transfusion and cord clamping issues. J Perinat Neonatal Nurs. 2012 Jul-Sep;26(3):202-17

310. Patel, S. Clark, EA. Effect of umbilical cord milking on morbidity and survival in extremely low gestational

age neonates. Am J Obstet Gynecol. 2014 Nov;211(5):519.e1-7

311. American College of Obstetricians and Gynecologists. Timing of umbilical cord clamping after birth. Committee Opinion No. 543. American College of Obstetricians and Gynecologists. Obstet Gynecol 2012;120:1522–6.

312. McAdams, RM. Time to implement delayed cord clamping. Obstet Gynecol. 2014 Mar;123(3):549-52

313. Bayer, K. Delayed Umbilical Cord Clamping in the 21st Century: Indications for Practice. Adv Neonatal Care. 2016 Feb;16(1):68-73

314. Raju, TN. Timing of umbilical cord clamping after birth for optimizing placental transfusion. Current Opinion of Pediatrics. 2013 Apr;25(2):180-7

315. Gupta, R. Ramji, S. Effect of delayed cord clamping on iron stores in infants born to anemic mothers: a randomized controlled trial. Indian Pediatr. 2002 Feb;39(2):130-5.

316. Emhamed, MO. van Rheenen, P. Brabin, BJ. The early effects of delayed cord clamping in term infants born to Libyan mothers. Tropical Doctor. 2004 Oct;34(4):218-22.

317. Strauss, R. Mock, D. et al. A randomized clinical trial comparing immediate versus delayed clamping of the umbilical cord in preterm infants: short-term clinical and laboratory endpoints. Transfusion. Author manuscript; available in PMC 2010 Jun 11.

318. World Health Organization. Optimal timing of cord clamping for the prevention of iron deficiency anaemia in infants. http://www.who.int/elena/titles/full_recommendations/cord_clamping/en/

319. Moore, D. MacDonald, N. Preventing ophthalmia neonatorum. Can J Infect Dis Med Microbiol. 2015 May-Jun; 26(3): 122–125.

320. Schaller, U. Klauss, V. Is Crede''s prophylaxis for ophthalmia neonatorum still valid? Bulletin of the World Health Organization, 2001, 79(3)

321. Lund, RJ. Kible, MA. Et al. Prophylaxis against gonococcal ophthalmia neonatorum. A prospective study. South African Medical Journal. 1987 Nov 7;72(9):620-2.

322. Ali, Z. Khadije, D. Et. Al. Prophylaxis of ophthalmia neonatorum comparison of betadine, erythromycin and no prophylaxis. J Trop Pediatr. 2007 Dec;53(6):388-92

323. American Academy of Pediatrics. Controversies Concerning Vitamin K and the Newborn. This policy is a revision of the policy in 112(1):191 Pediatrics May 1993, VOLUME 91 / ISSUE 5

324. Gopakumar, H. Sivji, R. Rajiv, PK. Vitamin K deficiency bleeding presenting as impending brain herniation. J Pediatr Neurosci. 2010 Jan-Jun; 5(1): 55–58.

325. National Institutes of Health. Vitamin K. Fact Sheet for Health Professionals. https://ods.od.nih.gov/factsheets/VitaminK-HealthProfessional/

326. Iioka, H. Akada, S. et al. A study on the placental transport mechanism of vitamin K2 (MK-4). Asia Oceania J Obstet Gynaecol. 1992 Mar;18(1):49-55

327. Koppe, JG. Pluim, E. Olie, K. Breastmilk, PCBs, dioxins and vitamin K deficiency: discussion paper. Journal Royal Society of Medicine. 1989 Jul; 82(7): 416–419.

328. Thijssen, H. Drittij, M. Et al. Menaquinone-4 in breast milk is derived from dietary phylloquinone. British Journal of Nutrition, Volume 87, Issue 3 March 2002, pp. 219-226

329. Merck and Co, INC. INJECTION AquaMEPHYTON® (PHYTONADIONE) Aqueous

Colloidal Solution of Vitamin K1.
http://web.archive.org/web/20070213093306/http://ww
w.fda.gov/medwatch/SAFETY/2003/03Feb_PI/AquaM
EPHYTON_PI.pdf

330. Page, G. Are There Long-Term Consequences of
Pain in Newborn or Very Young Infants? J Perinat
Educ. 2004 Summer; 13(3): 10–17.

331. Cheyney, M. Bovbjerg, M. et al. Outcomes of Care
for 16,924 Planned Home Births in the United States:
The Midwives Alliance of North America Statistics
Project, 2004 to 2009. Journal of Midwifery and
Women's Health. Volume 59, Issue 1
January/February 2014. Pages 17–27

332. Gilmartin, A. Ural, S. Repke, J. Gestational
Diabetes Mellitus. Reviews Obstetrics and
Gynecology. 2008 Summer; 1(3): 129–134.

333. Munro, IC. Hand, B. et al. Toxic effects of
brominated vegetable oils in rats. Toxicology and
Applied Pharmacology. Volume 22, Issue 3, July
1972, Pages 432–439

334. Sundararaman, PG. Sridhar, GR. Et al. Serum
chromium levels in gestational diabetes mellitus.
Indian J Endocrinology and Metabolism. 2012 Mar;
16(Suppl1): S70–S73.

335. Yin, J. Xing, H. Ye, J. Efficacy of Berberine in
Patients with Type 2 Diabetes. Metabolism. 2008
May; 57(5): 712–717.

336. Webb, S. Garrison, M. et al. Severity of ASD
symptoms and their correlation with the presence of
copy number variations and exposure to first trimester
ultrasound. Autism Research. August 2016

337. Newnham, JP. Evans, SF. Michael, CA. et al.
Effects of frequent ultrasound during pregnancy: a
randomised controlled trial. The Lancet. Volume 342,
Issue 8876, 9 October 1993, Pages 887-891

338. Ohlsson, A.   Shah, VS.   Intrapartum antibiotics for known maternal Group B streptococcal colonization. Cochrane Library.   10 June 2014

339. Wiley-Blackwell. Unnecessary induction of labor increases risk of cesarean section and other complications, study suggests. ScienceDaily. ScienceDaily, 6 March 2012.

340. American Pregnancy Association. Prolonged Labor: Failure to Progress. http://americanpregnancy.org/labor-and-birth/prolonged-labor-failure-progress/

341. Kingma, E. Improving Our Thinking. J Association for Improvements in the Maternity Services Journal. 2013, Vol 25 No 2

342. ACOG. Approaches to Limit Intervention During Labor and Birth. Number 687, February 2017

www.ingramcontent.com/pod-product-compliance
Lightning Source LLC
Chambersburg PA
CBHW060233290526
45789CB00001B/30